8 Profit Boosting Systems For Your Cosmetic Practice

How To Recession-Proof Your Practice,
Instantly Increase Your New Patients
& Grow Your Practice

LEGAL NOTICES

TABLE OF CONTENTS

PREFACE

If you have been sitting on the fence trying to figure out how you can use brand new marketing tools like Facebook, Twitter, YouTube, tablets and smartphones to get more patients into your practice, then the fact that massive success in your practice is closer now than it's ever been, should have you excited.

In fact, the current state of the economy in many local areas, which we find ourselves in is the perfect storm for doctors who are nimble and willing to ride the wave. However, taking advantage of this new economy comes with one requirement: You must take action *now*.

No more stalling, no more procrastination, no more day-dreaming about what it will feel like once you have a practice that runs smoothly and successfully without you. No longer can you straddle the fence, waiting and hoping that an ad rep strolls through your doors and magically solves all your marketing problems. See, the truth is that you are guaranteed to continue struggling if you are sitting back and hoping that you can simply buy the magic bullet.

What you hold in your hands is the ultimate step-by-step blueprint to take you by the hand and guide you through the danger-riddled, but rewarding journey of setting up marketing systems that will get new patients into your practice *today*.

In this book, I have compiled dozens of marketing strategies that successful doctors are using right now to consistently break sales and revenue records month after month. None of these strategies are untested theoretical ideas that haven't seen the light of day. Each marketing strategy and system has been painstakingly applied and leveraged to produce tens of thousands of dollars in profits each and every week, in every type of practice imaginable.

I have included the information you will want to know in order to effectively market your practice, but more importantly, I have included the information that you will NEED to know to avoid wasting tens of thousands on useless marketing strategies, ineffective advertising and expensive marketing mistakes.

The book you hold in your hands is unique in five major ways:

1. This book… is meant to be used as your personal guide to marketing your practice. There are plenty of books about running a practice or marketing, but this is the first book to extensively focus on marketing a practice in the ever-increasingly competitive market of aesthetic and plastic surgery.

2. This book… prepares you to become an expert at getting patients into your practice by empowering you with the exact information you need to know to market your practice. Nothing has been left out.

3. This book… breaks down all the vital parts of writing marketing messages that gets butts into your practice. It is not just a few scattered pages about marketing online, ads, training staff and so on. This book gives you the birds-eye view and then swoops down for an in-the-trenches inspection of each piece of the marketing formula.

4. This book… hands you the keys to unlock every piece of knowledge and resource that you will need to successfully market your practice.

5. The strategies in this medical practice marketing book have been tested for the following eight types of practices:

   - Cosmetic/Aesthetic Practices
   - Plastic Surgery Practices
   - Med Spas
   - Dermatologist Practices
   - Ophthalmologist Practices
   - Physical Therapy Practices
   - Chiropractic Practices
   - Alternative Care Practices

After reading this one-of-a-kind practice marketing blueprint you will know:

1. How to use a simple piece of paper and a pencil to create marketing pieces that bring in thousands of dollars to your practice within five to ten days.

2. The easy way to setup marketing systems that run on autopilot and allow you to increase your profits by more than you've ever dreamed would be possible.

3. The security of consistent success because you'll finally be confident in yourself, as you have the knowledge, tools and resources to stabilize your sales, profits and personal income.

By investing in this book, you opened the door to an entire library of information about marketing your practice that will serve as guiding lights of inspiration, encouragement and sometimes an occasional slap on the wrist.

Lastly, in order to avoid a decades old debate, the titles doctor, physician, and practice owner may be used interchangeably for the sake of convenience in teaching the material in the book.

See you on the inside,

Jon Nare

CHAPTER 1

Marketing Success Foundation:
Developing The Mindset To Achieve
Massive Success In Your Practice

The first chapter is called marketing success foundation and this chapter is all about developing the mindset to achieve massive success in your practice. In this chapter, you'll discover why just focusing on small goals with low expectations like trying to cover payroll and make a little extra to save for retirement is killing your practice.

This chapter will also help you to overcome your doubts and self-destructive habits that are holding you back in your personal life and your practice success. I will also reveal the real secret behind the success of millionaire physicians and teach you how to leverage their success and use it to achieve what you want in your own practice. Lastly, we'll talk about the key areas in your practice that you must measure and track on a daily basis in order to know how well your marketing efforts are working for your practice.

However, the fact of the matter is that in order for you to have any level of success with the strategies discussed in this book, you have to first embrace the same mindset, beliefs, habits and goals of other successful doctors. The harsh reality is that without the right mindset, beliefs, habits and goals, unfortunately, you're destined to fail. There is no magic pill and nothing I can teach you here that will overcome poor habits, lack of discipline and self-doubt.

If you're serious about your success, then your real foundation and the true starting point for you is that you have to address what's going on between your ears– what your beliefs are, what your mindset is, what your habits are and what your goals are.

Tested And Proven To Work

The strategies and systems in this book work and they're not classroom theory or untested ideas. These strategies form the foundation for thousands of successful doctors right now, all over the country. The only thing that will stop them from working for you is your own mindset. That's why you need to first address what's going on between your own two ears.

Within the pages of this book, everything you thought you knew about marketing your practice will be challenged, pushed and pulled in different directions by the strategies and concepts in this book. Trust me when I say that's a good thing, because at the end of this book you will finally have a blueprint for marketing success in your practice and that's what matters.

How Bad Do You Want It?

Let me ask you this: How bad do you really want it? Are you tired of struggling? Are you tired of the empty days and your staff standing around in your practice with nothing to do for hours at a time?

In order to get the most out of this book, you have to look within yourself and answer the question of how badly you want real success in your practice. There will also be things in this book that will challenge your closely held beliefs. That's intentional, but at the end of the day it doesn't matter what your employees think. It doesn't matter what your "mother-in-law" thinks. It doesn't matter what the guy down the street thinks. It doesn't matter that you'll never win a most beautiful advertising award for your marketing pieces. It doesn't even matter if it strokes your ego or not.

All that really matters is that the strategies in this book will put money in your bank account and help your practice become more successful. <u>That's what this entire book is about.</u>

Speaking of Success

My definition of a successful practice is a practice that consistently generates a profit that pays you a very nice salary of your own choosing. It's a practice that creates a financially valuable asset that allows you to live the lifestyle that you choose to live and doesn't require you to work like a dog for it to operate successfully. That's my definition of a successful practice. Hopefully, that's what your definition sounds like too.

Now, here's what success is not: working yourself into an early grave because you're trapped in a practice for eighteen or more hours a day. It is not success if you are terrified to pick up the phone when it rings because it might be a bill collector. It is not success when you are going through multiple divorces because you're a nervous wreck and a stressed out jerk, or missing out on seeing your kids grow up because you're stuck at the practice for weeks at a time.

That is not success by any stretch of anyone's imagination. But that is exactly what many doctors experience. The reason for many of their struggles is due to the fact that they have not learned how to successfully market and operate their practice.

Let's be honest. Nobody buys or starts a practice with the intention of working 90+ hours a week, getting paid less than minimum wage, having their reputation publicly trashed by complete strangers while risking going broke every few months and facing a life of bitter poverty.

Nobody buys or opens a practice with that in mind. But that is essentially what has happened, thousands of times, all over the country to doctors.

See, it's one thing to say that you want real success in your practice, but it's an entirely different thing to actually make that success a reality. So, I'm going to give it to you straight and you'll never again wonder how the other guys are doing it. You'll know exactly how they're doing it.

Your True Practice Success Foundation

There are five major ingredients that you need to have in order to turn your practice around and become truly successful:

1. You must **think** like a successful doctor.

2. You must **believe** you can actually become a successful doctor.

3. You must **embrace change** as a necessary part of your path to success.

4. You must **set goals** like a successful doctor.

5. You must **model** the systems of a successful doctor.

6. You must **measure and track** key performance indicators like a successful doctor would.

Ingredients For Success

With all of this in mind, let's take a look at the 6 ingredients for success that you will need to address before moving forward.

1. **What You Think** - The 11 unique ways a successful doctor thinks about their practice that's different from a struggling doctor.

2. **What You Believe** - The seven things a successful practice owner believes about their practice that's different from a struggling practice owner.

3. **Embrace Change** - The top 10 ways successful practice owners consistently embrace change in their practice in order to succeed in this challenging economy.

4. **Set & Pursue Goals** - How a successful practice owner sets & pursues goals in their practice that's different from average practice owners.

5. **Model Success** - The top systems that successful practice owners model that allow them to consistently generate record revenues while working less and living a balanced life.

6. **Measure & Track** - The important key performance indicators that successful practice owners measure, track and improve that average practice owners barely even notice!

Let's take a closer look at each of these success ingredients.

Success Ingredient #1 – What You Think
The 11 Unique Ways A Successful Doctor Thinks About Their Practice That's Different From A Struggling Doctor!

Every breakthrough and success you'll have in your practice starts with a simple thought in your mind. Thoughts are the seeds that grow into sales, profits and revenues.

If you can change the way you think, you can change your entire life and your practice. But you need to guard your mind like your life depends on it, because in fact your life does depend on your mind. You can't be passive about what you're reading, watching and listening to. You must be a vigilant soldier of your mindset.

Successful Practice Owner Difference #1

Successful doctors think about the habits they need to develop in order to accomplish their big goals. The truth of the matter is that your habits will either serve as a springboard to your next level of your success or serve as a quicksand pit that keeps you stuck at the current level or brings you even further down.

These successful habits include things like:

- Attending practice marketing and management conferences on a regular basis.

- Investing in and reading books and practice improvement books on a regular basis.

- Weekly meetings with staff and employees to track and review goals.

- Bringing in subject matter experts to quickly implement solutions.

Successful Practice Owner Difference #2

Successful doctors read, watch and listen to things that support their belief that success is truly possible in every area of their practice. It's a proven fact that if you truly believe something is possible you tend to focus on the ways to make that possibility a reality.

Also, if you don't think something is possible, then you will tend to focus on why it can't be done. There are three stages of possibility thinking that people can either get stuck in or go through:

1. Thinking nothing is possible no matter what they do.
2. Thinking that something is possible.
3. Thinking that anything is possible.

So, here's the question you need to ask yourself...

*"When presented with a challenge, do I first think
of the ways I could succeed or the ways I could fail?"*

High achieving doctors are always looking for ways to get to the level of success that they envision in their mind.

The only real question for successful doctors is what they must change or do in order to get to the next level of success and is that how you view your practice?

Successful Practice Owner Difference #3

Successful doctors know that they'll never be successful if they don't master delegation. The top doctors have a very specific view of their role as the owner and what they should and should not be doing in their practices.

They spend their time developing new marketing campaigns, creating new lines of practice and adapting to constantly changing local market conditions.

They know the value of creating systems for interviewing, selecting and hiring new employees, managing staff and using standard processes and procedures for every area of their practice.

Successful Practice Owner Difference #4

Successful doctors know that they have to stay the course and completely implement new patient attraction strategies even if they hit a snag while implementing them. They are able to move forward with good plans and marketing strategies, even if they are afraid.

One of the big obstacles for most doctors is that they take one or more steps forward, but because they hit a few roadblocks or issues, they then become paralyzed by the fear of failing.

When most doctors feel that fear, they tend to give in and lose all the momentum they've gained instead of stopping and reflecting on what's truly going on in their heart and mind, which is what successful doctors do.

In some cases, successful doctors are able to even use the fear of failure to motivate themselves to take massive action instead of being frozen with fear.

Successful Practice Owner Difference #5

Successful doctors know that they have to try many ideas and tactics to get the results they desire. See, if you know the odds of you succeeding are ten to one then you also know that if you have ten attempts, you're practically guaranteed to succeed at least once. All you need is ten attempts to guarantee your success.

Successful doctors are able to control and manage their perception of the journey that they're taking on the road to their success. It doesn't matter if you think that the glass is half full or the glass is half empty... both are right. It just boils down to your perspective on this situation.

Successful doctors know that failure is just a stepping-stone on their journey to success. They experience temporary setbacks and then build upon it to prevent it from happening again. Then, they move forward again from there.

Successful Practice Owner Difference #6

Successful doctors know that they can quickly grow their practice to huge levels of profits by finding creative ways to co-partner with other groups and practices. There are literally dozens of local groups, practice organizations and practice's that would love to partner with you.

When you become the "practice of choice" for several local practices, you gain access to thousands of patients that you don't have to pay advertising costs to get. Yes, it might mean donating products and services at events occasionally, but the extra profits you generate will more than make up for that expense. Because at the end of the day, you can add thousands of prospects to your marketing lists and databases without paying thousands of dollars of marketing expenses.

Successful Practice Owner Difference #7

Successful practitioners are always thinking about the goals and desires that patients want. Generally speaking patients want:

- **No pain:** Most patients will do anything under the sun to eliminate current pain or avoid pain on their path to recovery.

- **No fear:** Patients usually have a lot of questions that are related to their situation and the treatment plan you put together for them because most patients are focused on what could go wrong.

- **No complexity:** Many practitioners lose many potential patients because they can't communicate treatment plans simply and clearly.

- **Options:** Patients want several options in order to feel empowered while choosing their treatment plan.

- **Respect and courtesy:** The good old days when patients took your word as gospel truth are long gone. Patients are more informed than ever and need to be treated with respect.

Successful Practice Owner Difference #8

Successful doctors create and maintain standards for themselves and their employees so that they can consistently deliver excellence as their practice grows in size. The key is to clearly define what performance standards you need and then hold everyone accountable to meeting or exceeding those levels.

The standards that successful doctors develop and implement are then used as part of their advertising and marketing campaign to help them stand head and shoulders above their competitors.

Developing and implementing high standards in your practice sets you on the path for tremendous success as your practice grows.

Successful Practice Owner Difference #9

Successful doctors deliver an almost unbelievably high level of service that can rarely be matched. Successful doctors have a burning desire to serve their patients. They always focus on delivering a high level of service.

These doctors know exactly why people should choose their practice and are able to tell their prospects in clear terms. They rarely argue with a patient over an incorrect or mistaken order. The successful doctor knows what's really at stake in that transaction.

The successful doctor is always testing new products, services, vendors and combinations of all of them in order to continuously raise the standard of service in their practice.

Successful Practice Owner Difference #10

Successful doctors embrace new technology and cutting-edge marketing strategies. If you're still depending on fliers, door hangers and television commercials, then you're likely a few months away from bankruptcy.

Successful doctors know that text message marketing, online marketing strategies and current marketing strategies bring hundreds of patients each month like clockwork. That's why you have to keep an open mind to any marketing strategy that can be applied successfully to your practice.

Yes, you must include proven traditional strategies – I am not saying you throw those out of the window. But you **MUST** layer new cutting edge strategies on top of that foundation. Doing so will undoubtedly begin to deliver more in return for you marketing dollars.

Successful Practice Owner Difference #11

Successful doctors are always thinking about ways to remove all obstacles for attracting new patients, retaining current patients and following treatment plans.

They are intensely aware of the major barriers from a patient's perspective:

- Time
- Money
- Spouse or significant other
- Financial veto holder
- Societal beliefs (influence of others)
- Treatment outcome
- Fear (past experience, past imagined experience, current fear)
- Don't see, hear, or feel a need
- Too many choices
- Expectations (What will I look like? How will it work? How long will it last?)
- Psychological issues

<u>Success Ingredient #2 – What You Believe</u>
The Seven Things A Successful Practice Owner Believes About Their Practice That's Different From A Struggling Practice Owner

Your belief systems go hand-in-hand with your success mindset. They are inseparable. Many doctors have been one strategy or tweak away from success, but they stopped believing so they never experienced the level of success they wanted.

Without your belief, the seed you've planted in your heart and mind will wither and die. If you don't believe, then it's no surprise that your employees, spouse and patients also don't believe.

Successful Practice Owner Belief #1:

"A marketing strategy can only be successful if I fully implement it and test it out for an extended amount of time."

No matter how great and awesome a marketing strategy is, the marketing strategy is only as good as the doctor who is implementing it. You've got to implement the entire strategy before you can see if it works for you. You have no chance of it working if you don't even try it.

Once you get a strategy implemented, you have to let it run for at least 90 days so you can see the results and change things to get better results. You should always start by testing any strategy you're thinking of doing on a small selection of your patients and if that works, roll it out to all your patients.

Successful Practice Owner Belief #2:

"If there is a marketing strategy that works in other practices, then it can work in my practice and in my market too"

While you may need to tweak or adjust the specifics of the marketing strategy, if it has been done in another practice in another market, it can be done in your market.

When a doctor says "It can't be done in my market" what that means is that they are saying they haven't found the right way to make it work in their practice and until you actually try an approach that worked in another practice, you will never know whether it can or can't be done in yours.

Successful Practice Owner Belief #3:

> **"It's always better to invest a week or two initially setting up a process, system or strategy so that I can profit from that work for many years to come."**

Successful doctors are true believers in doing the hard work once and benefiting from that hard work over and over again. Here's how it can go... you can continue to work 110+ hours a week and make $150,000 a year or you can put in 20 hours of work once and earn a high six figure income every year for the rest of your life.

Understanding that your income will not necessarily increase because you work more hours is always a tough concept for most doctors to accept, but it's true.

You have to get into the habit of focusing really intensely for short periods of time to get strategies and systems implemented and then you can just spend a couple of hours a week optimizing and tracking the results and making changes based on the feedback.

Successful Practice Owner Belief #4:

> **"As long as a marketing strategy generates patients, sales and profits, then it's not too expensive."**

You're an entrepreneur, so by default you're putting it all on the line which means you will always have a certain level of risk no matter what you do. Therefore, a marketing strategy is only too expensive if it doesn't return an acceptable profit.

Managing the risk of investing money in marketing for your practice can be easily done by investing small amounts on a scheduled basis and then tracking your results before investing more.

The truth is that any dollar you spend that increases your net profit is ultimately a dollar well invested. It's not too risky when you break your marketing investment down into smaller dollar amounts and track your results to see what's working.

Successful Practice Owner Belief #5:

"Having good equipment, great location and trained staff are no longer good enough by themselves. I need to carve out a special place in the hearts and minds of my patients."

In this new economy, the old practice success formula is no longer good enough to succeed. Yes, you still need good equipment, good service and a competent staff, but in this day and age of competition, you also need to focus on selling a unique experience.

To reach your highest level of success with your practice, you must have a consistent and enjoyable experience for your patients every time they visit your practice. Then, you must ensure that your staff consistently delivers that experience according to the systems and standards you've set in place.

Successful Practice Owner Belief #6:

"I must invest in attending conferences, books and hiring qualified experts to help me always improve my practice and stay on top."

You should make it a habit to attend at least one industry conference and one marketing conference a year. There you will find doctors who have been in your exact situation and have figured out great solutions to the exact problem you're facing. They'll happily share their knowledge with you.

You also have to make it your personal mission to buy up books and training books by industry experts so that you stay ahead of your competitors. Once you've uncovered a problem that you can't solve or if you want to reach your goals faster, then it's time to bring in the experts.

Successful Practice Owner Belief #7:

"The financial success of my practice is directly dependent on my ability to train, inspire and manage my staff."

Obviously you can't run an entire practice by yourself, so it's vital that you build strong teams of loyal, dedicated and committed staff that will carry out your vision. If you spend all of your time doing everything personally, then you'll never be able to reach the higher levels that you want.

Your staff must know their daily, weekly and monthly goals and be properly trained, supported and managed in order to reach those goals. You must have your systems and processes down to an exact science so that all team members know their goals and responsibilities.

<u>Success Ingredient #3 – Embrace Change</u>
The Top 10 Ways Successful Practice Owners Consistently Embrace Change In Their Practice In Order To Succeed In This Challenging Economy

One of the constant things in life and in your practice is CHANGE. Each day presents a different set of circumstances and a different experience for you, your staff AND your patients. That's why you must constantly track, measure and react to changes in your practice and marketplace.

By the way, it's completely natural to desire to resist change and seek stability in order to make sense of the madness. However, many practitioners fight change even when it's crushing their practice profitability and is driving patients away.

Change Philosophy #1: Successful practitioners accept the fact that change constantly happens.

The desires, goals and expectations of your patients, staff and marketplace are constantly evolving or changing. You can't swim against the current and expect to not get burned out. Accept it and flow with it.

In fact, if you ever get tired of dealing with change and feel as though you're done with change, you're done with everything. You are a few years (if that) away from disaster.

Change Philosophy #2: Successful practitioners anticipate change and plan to leverage it.

Your goal must be to embrace and flow with change and figure out a way to turn the tables to your advantage. However, it requires you to do more than just observe and/or complain that things are changing.

You need to find a way to ride the wave of change and harness it to improve your systems and increase your profits. Sadly, struggling practitioners seldom anticipate or figure out a way to leverage the change in a successful way.

Change Philosophy #3: Successful practitioners constantly monitor change.

In order to leverage change, you must be tuned in and aware of the changes in the first place. The reason why is so that you can get actionable information and make strategic decisions that allow you to continue to grow your practice. Your goal must be to run your practice by the numbers.

Most practitioners don't know:

- Current profit and loss figures
- Number of new patients generated daily, week or monthly
- Production numbers or overhead costs

Therefore, they can't recognize downward trends or alarming patterns that would help them fix and improve their practice.

Change Philosophy #4: Successful practitioners quickly adapt to change.

Success in your practice will hinge on your ability to quickly implement improvements to address changes. While you do need to properly evaluate an opportunity, you can't afford to give in to paralysis through analysis, which is so prevalent in the healthcare industry.

At the end of the day, it's rare that everything will be perfect before you take action. So, you need to be able to take action on strategies, improvements and systems as soon as you have a minimum viable concept.

Change Philosophy #5: Successful practitioners know that they must make the transition to being action-oriented instead of being analysis-oriented.

After all, you can't just continue to do what you are currently doing and expect to go to the next level or get a different result. If you want to take it to another level you have to do something different first. In most cases, in order to take it up a notch, you have to change everything.

More revealing is the fact that failure to grow is failure to meet your patient's needs. There is no other reason for lack of growth. Therefore, you can correctly conclude that if you were meeting your patients' needs and properly communicating that to people in your marketing, you would be growing.

Change Philosophy #6: Successful practitioners grow to enjoy change and take pleasure in transforming unpredictable change into growth.

Ultimately, because change will be constant, you must learn to embrace it and enjoy it. You cannot expect to build a successful practice in this economy if you don't enjoy the journey.

You must get the point where you enthusiastically seek a new way, a better system, to stay on top. Of course getting to that point will take deliberate work because not all change is inherently fun. However, embracing and learning to be inspired by change should be your goal.

The Change Litmus Test

You know you need to change things in your practice when you often find yourself saying things like…

"The economy or my situation will get better."

The harsh reality is that it may not necessarily get better for you, especially if you're not doing anything differently to "make" things get better. Also, if the last decade or so has been an aberration, it will never get back to the "good ole days".

"It's the poor economy or some other "external" problem."

Don't look for an external solution for an internal problem. Regardless of what the economy is doing or any other external situation that's effecting you, there is always a doctor just down the street that is thriving and growing under the same conditions. You need to be that practice.

"My circumstances are different."

This is usually followed by how they are doing everything right, but fail to see why everything is not working. If you are not growing, you are not meeting your patient's needs and you're not communicating to your target market how you can meet their needs. It's really that simple.

Fail to give patients what they want, when they want it, at a price they can afford, and you are guaranteed to fail.

"I just need to be patient."

You can't afford to just sit back and wait until things get better. You must actively seek and implement new and improved strategies and systems. You need to do something different. If you follow this flawed strategy, you will move patiently into a failed practice.

"Patients will come back soon."

Unfortunately, unless you do something to get them back, they'll likely never come back. It's tough to come to terms with that reality.

If they left your practice, then they've found someone else who takes their insurance, has more convenient hours, charges reasonable fees, offers services that you don't, addresses their issue (if possible) on the first appointment or finds ways to make treatment affordable.

Face The Music

There is no magic wand that you can wave to make any of the false assumptions I just listed go away. These "false assumptions" are limiting beliefs. The real problem is if you hold a limiting belief long enough, it becomes truth for you. Once it is truth, it holds you captive and prevents you from being able to see the truth of your circumstances. Break the chains.

<u>**Success Ingredient #4 – Set & Pursue Goals**</u>
How A Successful Practice Owner Sets & Pursues Goals In Their Practice That's Different From Average Practice Owners

Now that you have made up your mind, clarified your thinking, and strengthened your beliefs, it's time to know and set your goals. Here's how a successful doctor **sets goals** for their practice that's different from average doctors.

In order to set goals, you need to answer one question. This one question will serve as your guiding light towards a successful practice… and that question is very simple…

"Where Are You Headed?"

Many doctors float aimlessly from one cash crisis to the next cash crisis. That's a terrible way to run your practice and it's an even worse way to live. At a minimum, you need to have daily, weekly and monthly goals. The smaller goals that you set will serve as your road map to your bigger goals.

You see, knowing where you're headed will set yourself off in the right direction so achieving big goals should be firmly guided by your smaller daily, weekly, and monthly goals.

Do You Have Big Goals For Your Practice?

It's been proven time and time again that tiny goals will result in tiny results. That's why you can't settle for your practice having extremely slow days and weeks because of seasonal changes, off-peak times and down times.

You can't approach this as if you're just trying to cover your overhead expenses and save a little bit of what's left over for a rainy day fund. Then, take most of that little bit that's left over and use it to try and prove to your spouse that things are okay. Those are small tiny goals, and they give you tiny results.

On the other hand, chasing after big goals will result in you getting bigger and bigger results. Here's some big goals that are worth chasing:

- Having a consistent flow patients coming into your practice every day of the week that you're open.
- Consistently processing thousands of dollars a week in sales through your website.
- Offering services and products at premium prices and having your patients pay in advance.
- Being featured in your local newspapers and media regularly.
- Expand your practice through franchising or opening up different locations.

Aren't those great goals and great results? Honestly, which one sounds more like you? See, the fact is…

"You will become as small as your controlling desire; or as great as your dominant aspiration."

So, you become as small as your thinking, or as great as your big goals. Don't be afraid to chase greatness.

Chasing Greatness

The truth is that most great achievements in life are the result of thinking big and aiming high. Small goals put chains, restrictions and limits on your potential, but when you're working towards a big goal you barrel right through dozens of smaller goals by virtue of chasing that big goal.

However in order to become your very best and reach those big goals you have to think at a very high level in regards to your goals.

Success Ingredient #5 – Model Success
The Top Systems That Successful Practice Owners Model That Allow Them To Consistently Generate Record Revenues While Working Less And Living A Balanced Life

Modeling the proven systems and processes of other successful practices is the missing ingredient that most doctors are looking for. Imagine having the exact strategies, process and systems that other successful doctors have used to explode their profits or as ways to get more patients.

It's all there waiting for you—they've done the work for you. However, the profits are not in simply having the blueprint in your hand but the real gold, the real profit, the real breakthrough, lies in your ability to actually implement the strategies that are proven to work.

Don't Reinvent The Wheel!!

Don't fall for the classic mistake of thinking that you are the only doctor who doesn't have enough money for advertising or that you're the only one being crowded out by big corporations.

Every problem or challenge you have in your practice has already been faced and solved by other successful doctors. You just have to put their solution into action in your practice. The real issue will be in finding the solution, but since you've invested in this book, you already have many of the answers you have been looking for.

The Power of Modeling

You have to start using blueprints or roadmaps by other successful doctors and it will dramatically decrease the amount of time and money you waste. That's why it's so important that you attend conferences, events and invest in resources by other successful doctors.

In regards to the power of modeling others success, Tony Robbins wrote in his book **Unlimited Power**:

➢ Long ago, he realized that success leaves clues, that people who produce outstanding results do specific things to create those results.

➢ Modeling is the pathway to excellence... The movers and shakers of the world are often professional modelers—people who have mastered the art of learning everything they can by following other people's experience rather than just relying on their own.

➢ To model excellence you should be a detective, an investigator, someone who asks lots of questions and tracks down all the clues to what produces that excellence. Building from the successes of others is one of the fundamental aspects of most learning.

But, even when you find successful practice systems and processes to model, you will have to overcome the final hurdle.

The Hidden Pitfall of Modeling

The irony is that when most struggling doctors get to peek behind the curtain of successful practices, they're quickly bored and unimpressed with the proven systems and processes that million dollar practices are using.

They often complain that it seems too simple and easy. They can't get their heads around how simple it can be to achieve massive success in their practice. So, they go back to their practices and either never attempt the strategy or make it so complicated that they give up on it.

The Hidden Path To Success?

Most doctors incorrectly think that the road to success is hidden away, and if you could find it, it would be twisting, uphill, covered in fog, and full of pitfalls. Therefore many struggling doctors:

• Distrust obvious and straight forward answers to their problems

• Complicate simple concepts because we think the truth is too "common sense."

• Gravitate towards the secretive and mysterious because they believe that they hold magical alluring qualities.

Model Your Way to Success

Successful doctors know that their success is dependent on their ability to discover the simple but powerful things that they can consistently do to grow their practice. They know that the more complicated it is, the less likely their staff will be able to implement it consistently.

No matter how simple it looks, they do it and test the results and you need to do the same for yourself. After all, a small round wheel is not complicated but yet it revolutionized the world.

Success Ingredient #6 – Measure & Track
The Important Key Performance Indicators That Successful Practice Owners Measure, Track And Improve That Average Practice Owners Barely Even Notice!

It's a well-known fact among successful practice owner's that you can't improve what you don't measure or track. In successful practice's knowing the daily, weekly and monthly numbers is as common as putting on shoes. They wouldn't dare dream of drifting aimlessly from day to day without knowing their numbers.

However, struggling practice owners do exactly that. You must know all the important numbers in your practice in order to make the right decisions that patient to lasting profits.

Key Area #1: Attracting New Patients

Patients are the lifeblood of your practice. Without a consistent flow of LOYAL patients, your practice is slowly but surely going out of practice. You should have several marketing campaigns that are always bringing new patients to your practice.

It's important that you're tracking your numbers in your practice. At the most basic level, you should know the following two numbers:

- How many new patients you get each day?
- What ad or marketing message brought the patient in?

Key Area #2: Track Patient Lead Sources

This seems obvious, but many practice owners don't track how many of their patients are coming in from their various marketing efforts. If you don't know what's working, then you may be wasting a ton of money on things that don't work.

You should know exactly what marketing strategies are working to bring people through your doors. The best way to do this is by providing a tracking system that could consist of a coupon, unique code or phrase that a patient must bring with them in order to get the deal advertised on the marketing piece.

Key Area #3: Lifetime Value of Patients

Successful practice owners know the lifetime value of each patient that walks into their practice. This is important because it determines how much you can invest on marketing and advertising to get and keep your patients.

So, if on average a patient comes to your practice twice a month for an average of five years and spends on average $200 per visit, then their lifetime value is $24,000.

Keep in mind that we're talking averages here, so that means that on average every one of your patients is worth $24,000 to you over five years. Therefore, is it reasonable to invest $30-$50 per patient to get them to come back to your practice again and again? Heck yeah it is!

Key Area #4: Staff

It is virtually impossible to maximize your practice's sales potential without your staff performing at their best. Your staff training is just as important as any other part of your practice.

Here are the three main areas that you need to train on:

1. Recruiting - What kind of people do I have?
2. Training - What training needs do I have?
3. Management - What performance or accountability issues do I have?

Key Area #5: Technology & Tools

It will be next to impossible for you to succeed in this new economy if you are not embracing current technology and tools. However, the technology you use in your practice must always help you reach real tangible goals. Technology tools can include everything from computers and software to marketing systems.

The questions you must ask yourself are:

1. What new systems or tools do you need to add?

2. What current systems or tools do you need to improve or upgrade?

Key Area #6: Personal Education & Growth

Your personal education should be prioritized and invested in just like any other part of your practice. There are new marketing strategies and new technologies that can make a tremendous impact on the success of your practice, but you must stay current on the knowledge.

Without your own personal development, you won't have the skills and knowledge to sustain the growth in your practice. You need to ask yourself the following questions:

1. What knowledge do I need to learn?

2. What skills do I need to acquire?

If you're currently not measuring or tracking any of the key performance indicators I just covered, then it will seem overwhelming when you finally start. But, do it anyway. It's not about what's easy, but it's about what works.

Start with simple tracking sheets that are included in this book and add your own custom performance indicators to those. The sooner you start tracking, the sooner you can improve.

CHAPTER 2

New Age Marketing: The New Rules About Marketing Your Practice In This Economy

Unless you've been living under a rock, you've noticed that the economy has changed and that attracting a constant flow of new patients while keeping your existing patients happy is harder than ever before.

Have You Noticed?

Have you noticed that ads and promotions that worked in the good ole' days, don't do diddly-squat now? Or that they don't get many patients in now?

Have you also noticed how it's costing you more and more just to break even and you feel lucky for even doing just that? Have you noticed that new practices are opening up all around you and you're losing patients left and right? Have you also noticed that things like coupon books and Valpak just aren't working anymore?

Long story short, it's tough out here right now, but why is it so much harder now to get more patients for your practice than it was before? Well, let's look at the barriers that are keeping most independent practitioners from breaking through.

The Top 10 Reasons Why Doctors Are Struggling To Succeed In This New Economy

Success Barrier #1: The doctor and staff don't own the process of learning and applying proven strategies.

The sad truth is that most doctors don't want to manage their office, deal with staff or manage the finances. They just want to treat patients. That's noble, but it's a naïve perspective that will end in your untimely demise.

The truth is that the act of leadership cannot be delegated or ignored. Whether by omission or commission, every success and failure in your practice is your fault or responsibility. Remember that you hired the staff, set up the hours, bought the location, marketed or failed to market, fell short of inspiring your patients… in short you were responsible for everything.

If you want a different result, you have to ensure that every action you and your staff makes contributes towards its implementation.

Success Barrier #2: Owning a practice in a geographical area filled with patient demographics that don't allow for practice growth.

There are many areas in the country that make growth almost impossible. Many experts agree that once you drop below the doctor to population ratio of 1:2000, you have entered an area of diminishing returns. Meaning marketing is more difficult because every doctor is doing it, and every person is exposed to it. Fees are more competitive. Patients have more choices.

In this type of situation, everything and everyone has to be at the top of your game. There is very little wiggle room to make a mistake.

If this is the case, your expectations on growth, new patients, production, and overhead need to be realistic. Without moving your practice, you will struggle for the remainder of your career.

Success Barrier #3: Making decisions for your practice based on old demographics of your target market.

Even if the demographics in your town or zip code, seemed right to you in the past, they tend to degrade and change over time. Every neighborhood degrades; it changes demographics, race, and income levels.

As it does, you will often find that your practice does not reflect these changes. This means that you unintentionally lost touch with your target. In order to be poised for success, your practice, staff, and overall systems must reflect the community you practice in.

Success Barrier #4: Having the wrong practice positioning and growth strategy.

Any marketing and practice growth strategy can work somewhere. However, that doesn't mean that any strategy will work for your practice. For example, while the idea of a cosmetic or boutique practice appeals to most doctors, your practice location, your personality, charisma, and clinical skills may not be able to support it because the success of each type of practice is dictated by the demographics of the area you serve.

Don't be fooled into thinking that a boutique practice is the only stress free, high profit, low overhead, and higher quality, higher calling type of practice. Make sure your choice of practice styles is supported by your circumstances and patient demand in your target market. After all, trying to sell patients what they do not want is a sure-fire way to financial and practice failure.

Success Barrier #5: Not being positioned for growth and success.

Many practices have burned out doctors, marginal staff, and are coasting until retirement. That's not a formula for success. If you are about to invest your hard-earned dollars and go all in on your practice growth you need to be poised for growth.

You need to have the right staff, great location, healthy profits, good overhead, growing practice, and a fully-engaged doctor who is looking to make things happen.

Also, your entire office needs to have a "Whatever it takes" mindset because it takes an overwhelming commitment to growth, excellence, time, money, and energy to get to your next level of success.

Success Barrier #6: Thinking that your most important job is to simply treat patients.

Successful practices realize that treating patients, chasing payments, making phone calls, dealing with insurance companies, etc. are just things that you do while you're doing your real job. Your real job and the key to a successful growing practice is based upon your ability to "inspire" your patients and staff to new levels.

You may not know it, but the best practices with the greatest number of new patients hire for people skills and self-motivation, and train them to do everything else. People skills cannot be taught or trained. You either have it or you don't. This is why bonus systems don't effectively motivate a marginal staff. You need to hire motivated people and then train them. Keep in mind that Job #1 is INSPIRING your patients and staff.

—

Success Barrier #7: Not understanding and integrating "Consumerism" in your practice marketing and advertising.

Patients in this day and age are more informed, educated and want to have input at every level of their treatment plan. You must absolutely accept that the success of your practice is driven by the whims of a fickle public.

Patients vote with their feet, and if you are not getting your share, it is the consumer telling you that you are not resonating with them. In other words, the business model you are currently using is not working in your target market. You either change or continue to struggle.

If you consistently fail to meet the expectation of the consumer (being caring, compassionate, comparable in pricing, competent, confident, convenient, and able to do what they "want" rather than just what you think they "need"), then you are destined to have your practice fail.

Success Barrier #8: Not having the capital to invest in turning your practice around.

Every doctor needs to know how to handle money in a strategic and disciplined way. Without the money management skills or spending discipline, the margins are so close that there is little or no money to invest in coaching, marketing, or capital to grow your practice.

On that note, it's important to mention that one of the biggest causes of financial issues is caused when a doctor believes that buying every piece of new technology is the path to practice success.

Nothing could be further from the truth, and nothing will sink you more quickly financially than over-spending. It is not unusual to see these same struggling doctors spending $30,000 in a year for clinical courses but fail to produce $30,000/month in their practice.

Success Barrier #9: Believing something about yourself, staff or patients to be true that is not true. This is called a limiting belief.

A limiting belief is a thought or process that you have held or performed so long that it has become truth to you. Most often the belief is untrue, but because it is the only thing you have experienced, you hold it as truth and that creates a filter through which you view and take action on all things.

Imagine the effect of believing that: I'm terrible with finances, I can't be a good leader, patients just can't afford my fees, there are no good employees around here etc.

None of these are truths, however, if you hold the wrong limiting belief long enough to make it truth for you, it severely hinders your ability to inspire others, implement new ideas and embrace change.

Success Barrier #10: Feeling entitled to success because you've "put your time in", therefore you are owed success by the universe.

If you have been running your practicing the same way for more than ten years, you are probably not even in touch with the reality of running a small consumer driven practice. In fact, if you have been in the same location more than 10-15 years you are probably in the wrong location for growth. The reason why I say that is because demographics, competition, median household incomes, race, and educational levels always change with time. Failure to meet these changes creates a plateau, an increase in cancelations and no-shows, lower productivity, and fewer new patients.

Gone are the times of no competition, work whenever you want, and charge whatever you think you can get away with just because you've been practicing for a long time.

Success Barrier #11: Not consistently marketing for new patients or current patients.

If you're only marketing sporadically, then that's why you're getting sporadic results. In order for you to have a consistent flow of new patients, you must implement a well-engineered marketing plan. However, your marketing plan must be a systematic outreach program that is dictated by your area demographics. Also, it must include a compelling offer and urgency to act in order to incentivize patients to come in on your time table.

Don't settle for just getting by while blaming a poor economy that might or might not correct. Recessions separate the marginal from the great.

On The Other Hand…

While I just shared the major barriers to success for most doctors in their practice's, I also want to share with you the new rules about marketing your practice that are helping doctors and practices thrive and experience record growth in this new economy. These doctors have figured out what their target demographic wants and they give it to them.

These doctors know how to leverage new trends and technologies in order to get new patients.

In short, they have figured out the new rules that govern marketing and growing their practice in this new economy. Now, let's look at the new rules of growing your practice in this new economy.

New Rule #1 Of Practice Marketing

The patient has the only vote that counts. Period.

One of the biggest marketing mistakes doctors make is not understanding and addressing patient needs. Most doctors NEVER ask their patients for feedback about what they did or didn't like about their appointment each visit.

The biggest breakthroughs in your practice usually come from your patients, but you must get the information from them. Including but not limited to: knowing what motivates the patients to choose your practice over your competitors. You also have to know what's most important to them when choosing a practice.

You have to know these kinds of things in order to understand your patients and to let them know that they have an important role to play in your practice.

New Rule #2 Of Practice Marketing

You must test everything in your practice first in order to improve upon it. Instead of guessing, test it out in an ad or on a patient and get their feedback.

Don't underestimate how powerful this is. You must test every component of your marketing pieces. If they don't at least pay for themselves, stop doing it. By the way, the only way to test something is to require the prospect to take a specific action upon seeing the advertisement.

This is called direct response advertising or direct response marketing. It allows you to measure and track the effectiveness of all your marketing.

It requires the prospect or the patient in this case to bring a coupon or some kind of tracking mechanism into your practice so that you know what advertisement or marketing message brought them into your practice.

New Rule #3 Of Practice Marketing

Prospects need a unique, persuasive and compelling reason to choose your practice over your competitors.

Every patient always wants to know what's in it for them if they choose your practice over your competitors. Don't waste your time with the normal self-promotional and bragging image advertising. Nobody cares how many awards and things like that you've got in the past.

Your marketing message must be specific to your prospects needs, wants and problems. You need a unique selling proposition (USP) that tells people exactly why they should choose your practice over any and every available option to them, including doing nothing.

New Rule #4 Of Practice Marketing

Stop trying to attract anyone and everyone to your practice. You should only focus on attracting the best type of patients to your practice.

You must pick a specific type of patient that you want to target and then tailor a specific marketing campaign to that type of patient. In your practice marketing campaign, you should never try to list everything you offer.

Pick one thing at a time and focus on it. Not everyone will appreciate your products and services. That's a fact of life. That's why your ads need to be specific and compelling to draw a specific type of patient.

New Rule #5 Of Practice Marketing

Patients must enjoy both the services and experience of being a patient at your practice. Get one of these wrong and you're guaranteed to struggle.

When it comes to offering stellar service, you should start by making sure your staff isn't slow to offer help or being rude to patients, because if so, patients won't stick around to give you another shot – there are just too many options out there.

Don't compromise on quality and variety to lower the cost. If anything, have separate lines of products, services, procedures and treatment plans to meet the needs of every type of patient.

Also, don't ever compromise on giving the best patient service but you should always strive to give the best experience for your patients at all times. Finally, make it your mission to continually ask your patients about what they would recommend you do in order to improve your practice.

New Rule #6 Of Practice Marketing

You must take scheduled time away from your practice to improve and implement the things that are important to your patients.

In order for you to view your practice from your patient's perspective, you must take time to step away from your practice and look at it from a patient's perspective. The key is to step outside your own shoes and begin to come up with new and exciting ways to get more patients and get your current patients to continue to come back.

Scheduled time to improve and implement—this is the highlight of this new rule. You can choose to do it every 6 months or once every quarter, or you may take a day or two to look at your numbers, revenues, sales, inventory, and all the different things that you needed to look at. This will help you figure out the area where you are weak.

You need to discover all the things that are going to keep your practice successful and all the things that keep the balance in your life. And to do that, you need to take scheduled time away from your practice at least once every six months or once every quarter.

New Rule #7 Of Practice Marketing

You can't do everything all by yourself, because it dramatically limits what you're able to accomplish.

If it's only you, then when you run out of time, money, energy, ideas, etc., there's going to be nothing and nobody else to help you. Many doctors think that they can do things by themselves if only they work harder. I say, don't fall into the trap of working harder, but getting less and less results. For example, do you earn twice as much if you work twice as hard? No!

This is where the role of your staff comes. Your staff is very essential for your practice. You must get your staff properly trained and implement technology where it's appropriate to help you make dramatic increases towards your goals and results.

New Rule #8 Of Practice Marketing

Stop reinventing the wheel every single time because of a lack of effective systems.

If your practice is not built on proven systems that you can easily teach your staff, then all you really have is a job that requires you to start over from the beginning every single day. This means that you need a system for everything—a system for attracting new patients, for collecting their contact information and providing them with superior service, for turning first-time patients into lifetime patients and then getting them to refer others to your practice.

You need systems for all of these things because the thing about a system that's so great—the reason why you need it in your practice—is because you need to know that you need to approach your marketing systems the same way you approach your serving systems.

You need to have these marketing systems in place to collect information and to keep people coming to your practice because nothing happens until somebody buys something.

New Rule #9 of Practice Marketing

You must actively get reviews and testimonials from your past patients to provide third party validation of your practice.

We live in an age of social media where everyone is connected and very vocal about the things they love or hate. That is why you can't simply sit around and hope that people say good things about your practice.

You need to be proactive and get patients to open up about the things they liked and then document it so you can use it on your website and in your marketing. You accomplish this by having your staff hand out comment feedback cards with every purchase and give them a little script to say as well.

The whole point of this is that you want your staff to prompt your patients to write down their feedback. You may want to invest in hand held cameras where they can get the patient on camera and tell them to say something positive about their visit.

Do this and you'll see that over time, you could easily get a hundred to two hundred testimonials that you could use on your website. You could use them in your marketing. You could get these people to go to Yelp or any number of review websites and leave their comments and feedback which in turn get you more patients and get more people to come to your practice.

New Rule #10 of Practice Marketing

You must list your practice in every online practice directory and review website that your patients use online to find practices like yours.

Online directories are very important when it comes to using the internet to attract more patients. That's why you have to make sure that your practice is listed in all the relevant online directions with fully completed business listings filled with testimonials and reviews.

The best way to get these reviews and testimonials is to reward your patients with a benefit, bonus or freebie for posting their feedback. It works wonders. This has to become a regular practice in your practice.

You or your staff should be handing out feedback cards that encourage and reward patients for posting a review on specific social media websites and review websites. Be sure to ask the patients to email a link to their review on the specific website so that you can use it in your marketing.

New Rule #11 of Practice Marketing

Build your in-house database by collecting the contact details, birthday and anniversary date (if applicable) of every patient.

Building and using your own database is so important because it allows you to generate revenue at any time by offering the contacts in your database a new enticing offer or special pricing to boost your sales and revenues. Plus it allows you to get off the sales revenue roller coaster and control the sales flow in your practice. Secondly, your practice will no longer be held hostage by the high costs of traditional marketing strategies. Lastly, you can test out new ideas and strategies without having to spend thousands of dollars to get new patients.

Missed Opportunity…

Most doctors spend thousands of dollars trying to get the attention of a small percentage of people who may possibly come to their practice, but do little to keep in contact with past patients.

Practice Insurance

Building a list of past patients that you can market your practice to on-demand is your insurance policy against the revenue roller coaster most doctors have to endure. Your database should be filled with hundreds of past patients who you can email and send your promotional offers to any time you want.

Imagine the power of sending out an email, text message, postcard or letter on Tuesday and being booked solid or flooded with patients for the next two months from that one marketing effort. That's powerful. That's what having an in-house list of past patients can do for you.

So Don't Be An Average Joe

Don't be an average doctor. Don't spend thousands of dollars on advertising with newspaper, radio, television, postcards or letters then wish and hope the ad is good enough to attract new patients to cover the costs of ad and make a little profit only to end with them coming to your practice but never hearing from you again.

That's a tragedy that's replayed over and over in practices all across the country. You have to be smarter than this. You have to be more efficient and strategic about what you're doing.

Successful Practice Owners Know That Money Is In The List

For every successful doctor, the long-term and sustainable profits are in having a list of happy past patients to market your offers to. So if a person calls/walks-in/emails/visits your website or steps into your practice, then you **MUST** make a conscious effort get their contact information. If you fail to do that, you will likely lose that patient forever.

The Next Step… Track Your Leads!

Once you have the long list of happy past patients, the next step is to track everything about your patients. You need to track which coupon or offer brought them in, how many people come in with them, how they heard about your practice, what days the patients come in, and the cost per source and cost per patient. Track everything because you need to know what's working so that you can do more of it or improve on it.

By The Way…

While it's very important to capture the contact information of every person who contacts your practice, it's also important to create a separate list of past patients explicitly. You need things like: name, address, how much they spent, birthday, anniversary, and children's birthdays. You need all the things that will be important for you to know in order to send out a timely promotion to them.

By collecting your patient's information, you'll begin to see patterns with your prospective patients like:

- Where they live
- How much they spent
- What procedures and treatments they purchased
- What offer or coupon brought them in
- Birthday
- Anniversary

All of these things are very important pieces of information. Once you begin to even use your point of sale system or develop another system for collecting contact information from your patients, you will begin to see trends that you can then use and optimize and maximize to get more sales and get them to come back to your practice more often.

Once you get the hang of building your database, you may then proceed to the next level—targeting your patients.

The Next Level

By getting this demographic information, you'll be able to laser target your marketing and advertising to your ideal patient by using things like age, race, marital status, income, hobbies. You will have all the things that resonate with your target market because you have the right information.

Now, once you have your target patients and their contact information which you have gathered from your own database, the next key step to successful marketing is consistent follow up.

<u>**New Rule #12 of Practice Marketing**</u>

**You must send weekly or monthly marketing messages
to your patient database until they move or die.**

The only reason that in your marketing you should collect and track the contact information of your leads and past patients is so that you can follow up with them regularly and consistently, to get them to come back to your practice and tell others about your practice.

Consistent follow-up is probably the single biggest problem that doctors have. Without consistent follow-up, you leave everything up to chance and the whims and wishes of your patients. You can't chance that.

You need to make sure that every week you have marketing messages going out, whether it's an email or text message or post card, or some other things that you have going out to your patient database. This needs to be like clockwork (i.e. once or twice a week, a couple of times a month). It just needs to be consistent and regular.

New Rule #13 of Practice Marketing

You will train your staff on how to politely and naturally lead patients into choosing effective longer term treatment plans.

Patients in this new economy don't want to be aggressively sold anything, so you need to train your staff to be patiently helpful. Just because a treatment makes you more profit, doesn't mean that your staff has to be forceful about offering it to patients.

Train your staff to ask leading questions that get patients to reveal their true goals and desires and then your staff can guide them to a good choice that strikes an appropriate balance between treatment plan length, results the patient achieves and profit generated. This will ensure that your patients have a pleasant experience at your practice.

New Rule #14 of Practice Marketing

**You will embrace consumerism and make it
a part of all your marketing.**

This means you will give patients what they want, at a time they would like it, and at a price that fits their budget. It is not enough to understand that patients or consumers have a choice; you need to become that choice.

Your goal is to inspire them, exceed their expectations and become an expert of budgeting the treatment they need. All while being sensitive to the reality that time and trust will be the final deciders of whether or not they choose you.

New Rule #15 Of Practice Marketing

The success of your practice depends on you successfully marketing your practice to your target market.

Marketing your practice successfully requires you to have a well thought-out yearlong consistent marketing plan. Your marketing plan must utilize both internal and external marketing strategies and embrace consumerism through demographics. You must use all types of marketing because it is no longer possible to reach the public and compete with corporate run practices through just one media or outlet.

After all, you are competing against well-funded practices with better hours, more marketing, better locations, and systems to buy supplies cheaper and train their staff better. You need to do everything in your power to gain the advantage.

New Rule #16 Of Practice Marketing

You must constantly expand your expertise so that you can grow your revenue by expanding your services.

Many doctors love the concept of a boutique practice, however, why impose built-in limitations to your growth? By expanding your expertise, you can add services that would expand the productivity and range of patients you could attract.

That's why patients are flocking to corporate run practices. The corporate run have figured out that patients love being able to go to one practice for every service possible.

Most times you will find that with these new areas of expertise, you will find new technology that compliments its application. Technology that pays for itself is a great investment when you consider how it affects overhead and debt.

New Rule #17 Of Practice Marketing

Become an expert at helping patients afford what they need by creating custom payment plans.

You must make a concerted effort to both train and hire staff members that are experts in finding the correct financing solutions for various types of patients. It is no longer good enough to just point to the fact that you offer financing options; you have to find flexible financial arrangements for each patient.

Once again, this is an area in which corporate-run practices are winning. They know that patients are thankful and loyal when they've been given a payment plan that fits their budget. Coming up with payment arrangements that work for you and your patients will continue to be a challenge, but to succeed in this new economy, you will have to master this skill.

New Rule #18 Of Practice Marketing

Spend time to connect with your patient's needs regarding their insurance.

With a large percentage of the population having some form of insurance coverage, you can no longer afford to create barriers to treatment by assuming that they will continue to come to you as an out of network provider.

Insurance like so many other things (not being open the right hours, not starting treatment plans on the first appointment, or not having services, procedures or treatment plans that patients actually want) creates a barrier to entry into your practice.

You need to examine how your current policies and systems are preventing patients from saying yes. Start by studying in earnest every insurance plan and learn how to maximize the patients' benefits while optimizing reimbursements.

Thoughts On All These New Rules

I realize that the new rules I just covered seems like a lot. However, the truth is you must approach marketing and running your practice in a new way because you're in a very different economy from twenty, ten or even five years ago.

In order to succeed in this new economy, you must do things very differently than you've done in the past. That's your new reality.

This Is About New Beginnings

When I talk about new reality, it means new beginning. New things like:

- New Marketing Strategies
- New Overall Focus For Your Practice
- New Direction For Your Practice
- New Training For Your Staff
- New Outlook On Your Marketplace
- New Staff

This Is About Building New Habits

When you do new things, you should also start to build new habits. You have to learn from your competitor's successes and failures. Develop a new habit of **asking and listening** to your patients. Learn to take the best ideas from different industries and apply them to your practice.

It's Time To Face The Music…

The market's changed. The desires and expectations of patients have changed. The economy has changed. The question is…

>> Why haven't you changed? <<

The Old Way:

You're still doing things the old way if you're being a slave to your practice and you commonly work 14-18 hours a day. You still haven't changed, if you were forced to submit to every whim of every Tom,

Dick and Harry that comes into your practice because you're desperate for money.

You are still doing things the old ways if you try to sell anything and everything that you can because you're trying to be a one-stop shop practice. You're still in the old way if you were wasting tons of money on image ads that brag about how great your practice is.

The New Way:

- You're in the new era if there are new patients "finding" your practice every day online.

- You have developed a new way of knowing exactly what ad or marketing effort generated every patient who visits your practice.

- You are adapting to the new era if you are collecting your patient's contact information so you can notify them of your practice's specials, or you are now using technology to attract new patients 24/7.

In this new era, you delegate as much as possible so you can spend your hours working on improving your practice instead of working for your practice.

It's about enjoying your life and having greater peace of mind knowing you have leveraged the best system to help you get the best possible result.

The One Thing…

What's the one thing that will determine whether or not your practice succeeds or fails in this new economy? Is it product quality? Is it patient service? Or is it good staff & support team? Is it because you have the lowest prices on the block or the best location in town?

WRONG!

"Your ability to consistently attract new patients and convert them into loyal patients. That is the **number one determinant** *of your real practice success. – In other words MARKETING!"*

The Secret To Success

"The sooner you become the marketer of your practice, instead of the doer of your practice, the faster your income and practice will grow!"

What Is The New Definition of Marketing?

Marketing is anything that you would do or can do to get patients AND keep patients. Period.

Everything is marketing…and marketing is everything to your success.

Marketing is using…

- Display ads
- Television Commercials
- Newsletters
- Websites
- Flyers
- Postcards
- Yellow Page Ads
- Letterhead
- Practice Cards
- Signs
- Billboards
- Loyalty programs
- Every interactions with patients and prospects
- **<u>EVERYTHING IS MARKETING!!!</u>**

Everything that you can do to either get patients or to keep them loyal to your practice is marketing!

The Light Comes On…

When you realize that **<u>"everything is marketing…"</u>** your practice, and the opportunities to market your practice, looks totally different to you. You see obvious mistakes, then you consider how your patients or potential patients might view situations, events or documents.

You will see missed opportunities and a ton of opportunities for improvement when you begin to look at this as everything-has-a-potential-to-be-a marketing message.

No Spray and Pray...

However, **ALL** marketing strategies **MUST** be held accountable to produce profits. This means that you must know the effectiveness of each ad, coupon, letter, flyer, postcard, TV commercial etc.

Your goal is to create a marketing system that's predictable and able to be duplicated month in and month out. In order to reach that goal, you should be able to know the exact ad that brought every patient into your practice.

Bring Friends, Or Else...

Once you are able to create and duplicate a marketing system, your next focus should be on the return on investment.

Every dollar that you spend must come back to your bank account with *at least* 5 new friends to join him. When done correctly, there is no better investment in your practice than marketing. Everything else is a cost. You must know your return on investment (ROI) at all times by using direct response marketing.

Direct Response Marketing

Direct Response Marketing is a marketing strategy designed to generate an immediate response or immediate action from a prospect, where each response (and purchase) can be measured, and attributed, and connected to individual advertisements.

Why Direct Response Marketing?

There are a lot of reasons why you should opt for direct response marketing. First, direct response marketing is personal, specific, clear and simple. Secondly, it's two-way communication because it gets your marketing message out but it also lets you know exactly what marketing message got people in to see you.

In other words, direct response marketing allows you to know exactly what the value of a patient is, because you know exactly what marketing piece brought them in.

Make It Plain & Simple

You start transitioning to direct response marketing by understanding the benefits your patients want and then offer that to them in your ads.

Communicate these benefits in an attention-grabbing, compelling and motivating manner. Next, you need to make an offer that has universal appeal to your defined target. Be sure to make a soft offer that is non-threatening for potential buyer to respond to.

Make it easy and non-threatening for first-time patients to step into your practice and enjoy their first meal. Some doctors offer huge discounts or free coffee to break the ice and create the momentum. Then when you have the momentum, start to implement tracking mechanisms in your ads that you can test while tracking.

The Direct Response Difference

Using direct response marketing makes your ads and marketing messages much more effective. It starts with an attention grabbing headline that makes a bold and simple to understand claim, promise or offer. The headline qualifies who the remainder of the message/ad is written for. This kind of marketing has ONE clear and simple goal to get the prospective patients to step into your practice to get what they want and need.

It also presents a clear call to action. For example, "Tell the person at the front desk this phrase…", "Go to this website…", "Bring this coupon in on this date…" etc. Direct response marketing allows you to know the true value and worth of each and every patient.

Coming Up Short

One of the reasons why many doctors have problems with their marketing strategies is because they don't know the value of their patients and therefore shy away from investing the needed amount of money into marketing to get that patient. When you use direct response marketing and keep an up to date and accurate database of your past patients, you can accurately measure the value of every patient for their lifetime. This is called the lifetime value of a patient.

Lifetime value is how much revenue a patient or patient will bring into your practice during their lifetime of dining at your practice.

Lifetime Value Of A Patient

Lifetime value is how much a patient is worth to you. Why is that important? Because that helps you make strategic decisions about your marketing budget to get a new patient and it allows you to forecast ahead.

Here's how it works:

- Take your last 12 months collections and divide that by the number of new patients you got that were NOT referred or reactivated.

- Let's say you collected $450,000 last year and had 285 total new patients.

- By dividing $450,000 by 285 you get an annual patient value of $1,578.95. That's how much you collect from the average patient over the first year.

Therefore, on average, you can theorize that if you wanted to invest $100 to get one patient, you'd still be very profitable.

Lifetime Value Of A Patient

The real power and breakthrough in your practice will occur when you harness the knowledge of the lifetime value of your patients and use it to implement direct response marketing in all your advertising.

It All Starts To Make Sense

When you realize that the lifetime value of your regular patients is $6,000 or more over a five year period, giving away a free gift or discount is just a drop in the bucket. Now, all of a sudden you get excited about getting as many of these patients as possible.

Plus, it starts to make sense to consistently run all the marketing strategies you can afford because you know they each represent $6,000 to you in the long term and when you can show your staff that those coupons and inexpensive little gifts actually represent a huge chunk of sales and revenue, they'll finally get the big picture.

CHAPTER 3

Patient Attraction Systems:
How To Stand Head And Shoulders Above
Your Competitors While Attracting
The Most Profitable Patients

In this chapter you'll discover the easiest and quickest way to motivate the right type of patients to choose your practice. We don't want to fill your practice with cheap skates. That's not the purpose of this book. We're going to talk about how to create a persuasive and compelling marketing message to your target audience that results in profits.

I'm going to teach you how to make your practice stand head and shoulders above your competitors and how you will always stick out in your patient's minds by giving you proven formulas you can use to make you the clear and obvious choice to your ideal patient.

You're also going to learn the real truth about the secret way to get people to try your practice the first time so that they can get hooked and give you an opportunity to get them as patients.

But first, can you answer this very important question…

"Why should a patient choose your practice over any other practice and over any other option that's available to them, including doing nothing?"

Trouble In Paradise…

If you struggle to come up with an answer to that question, that explains why you are not consistently attracting and retaining your patients! After all *you* don't even know why they should choose your practice.

Stand Out Or Sit Down

You will always struggle to attract new patients and retain your existing patients if you don't have a compelling reason for them to consistently choose your practice over your competitors.

You may be able to scrape by waiting for walk-in traffic or maybe an ad you run every now and then, but you'll never get to high levels of success without a unique hook, something that speaks to your target prospects and motivates them to get off their couch and come into your practice.

The "thing" or "combination of things" that makes your practice stand out in your patients mind is called your unique sales proposition (USP).

A unique sales proposition can make all the difference for your practice. It's the one thing that you have that you become known for or that people associate with your practice.

It is also known as…

- Point of difference
- Unique Perceived Benefit
- Unique Selling Point
- Extra Value Proposition
- Competitive Advantage

Regardless of the name you call it, it's the same thing… it's that thing that your practice can do, or the experience that you can provide, that is your uniqueness.

Dead In The Water

Not being able to distinguish yourself from your competitors is a curse that will haunt you for as long as your practice is open until you address it.

A practice with no USP is always at the mercy of the market place, cheap patients or cut throat suppliers. Also, a practice without a USP is also ripe for the picking for knockoffs, local competitors and big chain competition. After all, they do the same thing that everyone else does.

Therefore, you need to do something that makes your practice unique and makes it stand out in your local marketplace. When you don't have a USP and your supplier prices or operating expenses go up, then your profits always go down because you don't give your patients any reason why they should pay you one penny more than they're paying you now.

You're In Control

An effective USP gives you the power in every area of your practice. You get to pick the exact patient you want. You get the power to set your own terms. You get the power to charge higher prices. You can dictate your terms to your suppliers because you do higher volume. You get to choose your busiest days or down time.

In short, your practice is back under your control because you have something that can't be duplicated. You have something that no one else can do the way that you do it and so you can demand a premium for it.

It Gets Even Better

A really good USP does more than just get you patients. It also sets the strategic direction for your practice. It lets everyone know what to expect from your practice. Your USP is not simply a marketing or advertising "thing".

A compelling USP is more than a headline at the top of your ads. Your USP is the backbone of your practice. A good USP is more valuable than any marketing gimmick, newspaper ad or flyer. In essence, it's your entire practice in a nutshell.

Effective USP Essentials

There are several components that you need to include in your USP to make it stand out on your patient's mind.

First, each advertisement must make a relevant appealing offer to the patient or patient. It can't just be shallow words or purely advertising. The advertisement must tell the patient that if they come to your practice, they will get this specific result or benefit.

Secondly, the offer you're making in your advertisement must be something that your competition cannot or does not or is not willing to offer. It must be unique in some way that makes it stand out in the minds of your target market. The offer must be so compelling that it can get people to get up off their couches right now and come to your practice today.

However don't make the mistake of trying to compete on low price alone. As you build better USP's and you get a proven track record for delivering on your USP, you should be raising your prices.

How Many USP's Do You Need?

There are two groups of USP's that you will have to create:

1. **USP Group #1:** This is your overall practice USP that focuses on the general experience or expectations a patient should have when they reach your practice.
2. **USP Group #2:** This is the USP you create for each specific ad, special, promotion, product or service that you offer.

Yes, you need both types of USP's for your practice to stand out in the minds of your target market.

Bad & Ineffective USP's

While a good USP can help your practice consistently break sales records and grow profits, a bad USP can repel the exact patients you're trying to attract.

Here are some examples:

- Been in practice X amount of years.
- We have the cheapest prices for _____.
- We offer every type of procedure.
- Satisfaction guaranteed.
- We are the best s_____ in our town.

When you use any of those in your marketing all your prospects hear is a bunch of empty platitudes.

Overall Practice U.S.P's That Sell

Let's take a look at some examples of industries that have USPs that have sold billions of dollars in products and services to their target markets:

- Fed-Ex: *When it absolutely, positively has to be there next day.*

  When you had a high priority document that you needed to get somewhere overnight, you probably chose Fedex.

- Raymour & Flanigan: *3 Day delivery guaranteed.*

  They have guaranteed delivery of your furniture in 3 days or less. They were the first furniture retailer in New England to offer 3 day delivery, so if you needed it fast, you choose Raymour & Flanigan.

- Domino's: *Delivery in 30 minutes or its free.*

  If you were hungry and needed pizza fast, then you chose Domino's. Notice that they didn't say good pizza. They're just talking about 30 minutes and you have hot pizza.

What Do All Those USP's Have In Common?

All of the example USP's above were in very high competition industries. They spoke to their target market with their USPs. Most target a niche within a niche.

All were regular, boring products like furniture, mail delivery, and pizza. There was nothing special about the industries on the examples I just gave you. They were precise enough to echo the prospects' thoughts.

For example, if you're sitting at home and you wanted something to quickly eat without cooking, you chose Domino's. They were guaranteeing either it's 30 minutes or it's free.

USP's work because they address the biggest objection or fear to buying. If you were in the market for furniture and you came across Raymour & Flanigan's ads, you definitely paid attention. After all, there's nothing worse than paying thousands of dollars for furniture and having to wait when you have your in-laws coming into town but you have to wait six months when you wanted it in 3 days or less.

Each of the example USP's also promise to solve one problem that the prospect will pay to have solved. If you wanted something overnight and you were willing to pay that premium to Fed-Ex to get it there overnight, that wasn't a big problem. They all include the dominant emotion driving the prospect. You wanted it fast and you needed it quick—dominant emotions.

It's unique enough to be easily memorable. Most doctors don't have the guts to make strong guarantees. It's just what it is. But if Fed-Ex did it… if Domino's did it… if Raymour & Flanigan did it, you can do it too!

You just have to be creative and you have to take the time to make sure that you can deliver on your promise. It's a worthwhile investment of your time.

CHAPTER 4

Million Dollar Marketing Messages:
Marketing Messages That Consistently
Fill Your Practice With High Quality
Leads And Eager Prospects

Most doctors waste tens of thousands of dollars on ads, flyers and marketing strategies that never have a chance of being successful. Sadly, the reason why their ads and marketing don't work is because the doctors are allowing ad reps to create the ads and offers.

Also, in most cases, the ad reps only recommend extreme discounting as the only thing that's working in today's market. Nothing could be further from the truth.

If you had to take a guess, who do you think knows the patients and at your practice better than you and your staff? Nobody does! That's why you, along with the input of your staff who understand your vision and patients, should be the ones creating your ads, offers and marketing messages.

The Necessary Ingredient

As a doctor, you must know how to create simple but effective marketing messages that attract the right type of patients to your practice. There is no excuse for you, as the doctor, not knowing how to create marketing messages that attract patients. If you don't do it and if you don't know it, who does know it and who will do it?

The truth is that being able to create marketing messages is just as important as any other skill in your practice. In fact, without knowing how to create marketing messages that consistently attract patients, you're always just one bad month, quarter or year away from going out of business. So stop living on the edge. You definitely need to know how to write simple but effective marketing messages.

It's Not Rocket Science

You don't have to become a professional writer or a graphic designer in order to create great marketing resources that generate patients. You don't need a fancy computer, college degree or expensive software to make good ads for your practice. Some of the best ads and offers were written using a pen and a napkin.

You just have to be willing to spend a few hours a week writing down new and different ways to get the attention of your target market and your past patients.

It's no different than coming up with treatment plans for all the various patients who come through your practice doors.

What Is A Marketing Message?

A marketing message is any ad, flyer, email, tweet, postcard or anything else you can use to communicate your offer to prospective patients or to past patients that encourage them to come back to your practice.

Coming up with a good effective marketing message is not some complicated, confusing thing that will take you twenty years to learn. If you can talk to people, then you can write effective marketing messages for your practice.

Simply put, writing a marketing message is your ability to put on paper what you've already been saying to friends and family to get them to come to your practice.

The Core of The Problem

Without having a proven system for creating good offers, ads and marketing messages, most doctors have little to no chance of succeeding long term. In fact, most doctors are doing their marketing completely backwards.

- They are advertising to the worst possible target markets.

- In the most expensive and least effective places.

- Making the worst possible offers.

- To people that couldn't care less.

- While ignoring the best possible patients!

Let's break it down and examine each marketing mistake.

Marketing Problem #1:

Advertising to the worst possible target market.

If you ask the average doctor who is his target market, he would answer you by saying that anybody with a certain condition, disease or problem. However, the fact of the matter is that only a certain percentage of the population in your area will ever be in the market for the procedures and treatments you offer.

The worst possible target markets are people who don't have insurance, bad credit, no money and don't have a desire to address their ailment or subscribe to a better lifestyle. It doesn't mean that you can't help them, you can and should. However, you can't run a profitable practice focusing on them.

It's ridiculous to think that every single person will like what you're offering. Yet, most doctors think everyone is their target market. That's completely wrong and that's why they waste thousands of dollars trying to market to everybody.

Marketing Problem #2:

Advertising in the most expensive and least effective places.

The second big marketing mistakes committed by doctors is advertising in the most expensive and ineffective places. There was a day and a time when your local yellow pages, newspaper, radio and television stations would get you all the patients you would ever need. That day has come and gone.

Now, the big four: yellow pages, newspaper, radio and television are little more than a waste of money for the majority of doctors. That's not to say that you wouldn't get any patients from marketing in them, but there are places to advertise that are less expensive and more effective. At the end of the day, you shouldn't be advertising anywhere that your ideal target market doesn't hang out.

So, Where Should You Advertise These Days?

In today's digital age, there are more places to advertise than ever before, but the least expensive and most effective marketing strategies are the ones that only target your ideal patients.

For example:

- Sending an email or text message to a past patient for your "past patient only" offer costs less than one cent each.

- Showing your ads on Facebook for less than $5-$10 per day to people who have shown an interest in the product or services your practice offers.

- Having your ads and/or website show up in Google when people in your area search for the product or services your practice offers.

- Capturing every person who shows interest in what you offer and showing up on whatever website they go to… keeping you front and center in their mind until they are ready to buy.

There are dozens of ways to only invest your marketing dollars with people who have already demonstrated that they would be a good fit for your practice. That's where you should be advertising in this day and age.

Marketing Problem #3:

Making the worst possible offers when you're advertising.

The worst possible offer is an offer that doesn't persuade your ideal target market to come into your practice or an offer that attracts the type of patients that you don't want.

While you should give all patients that walk through your door the same quality of service, you must acknowledge that many people who walk through your door are not your ideal patient.

It doesn't make you a bad person. It just makes you a smart doctor and marketer. Your goal is to attract your ideal target market with your offers.

Also, most doctors think that lowering their prices is the only offer that will work to get new people in the door but that's not true. More importantly, if you only use price discounts to get patients then you are training your patients to only buy when you are lowering your prices. That's a terrible and dangerous way to run your practice

So, What Are The Best Type of Offers?

Your offer is the heart and soul of your marketing efforts. Without a good offer, nothing you say or do in your ad will matter. Therefore the best type of offers are the offers that attract your ideal target market and get them to come in and spend more money, visit more frequently and generate more referrals.

What Offers Does Your Target Market Want?

Every type of target market will respond differently to various offers. Your goal after you figure out your target markets is to begin to come up with offers that appeal to them in a persuasive way.

The best way to figure out what your patients or clients want is to consistently ask them and to look at your past sales receipts. If you're completely lost about how to create offers, then look at your receipts for what your patients are already purchasing.

That will give you crystal clarity about what they value or want more of. This will become easier for you to do as you begin to practice this more often.

Marketing Problem #4:

Advertising and marketing to people that couldn't care less.

No matter how great your procedures and treatment plans are at your practice, there are people who will never come to your practice. You shouldn't waste one penny advertising to those types of people because it's a huge waste of resources.

Most doctors will never even acknowledge that these types of people exist. They mistakenly think that everybody with a certain condition, disease or issue is their potential target market. For example:

- If you have a practice that focuses on cosmetic surgery, you may want to target a specific group such as individuals between the ages of 35-65 with incomes of over $100,000 for certain cosmetic procedures.

- If you decide to target your chiropractic services toward all the baseball teams in your area, then you will want to be visiting team workouts and games for observation, treatment follow up, holding injury prevention clinics and physicals.

So, Who Would Most Enjoy Your Practice?

Through technology, you can laser target your marketing messages to people who have either expressed their interest in the exact type of product or service you offer or they've shopped at a practice like yours before.

There's no reason why you should waste thousands of dollars on mass advertising methods where 98% of the marketing messages are sent to the wrong people.

Especially when ad platforms like Facebook allow you to target your ads to people who have stated that they like the exact type of products, services and experience your practice offers.

There are dozens of strategies that allow you to only focus on people who would be most likely to shop at your practice. That's what you should be doing.

Marketing Problem #5:

Ignoring the best possible patients!

Most doctors spend all of their marketing dollars trying to get new patients, but spend little to no money on the best type of patient.

And just so we're clear: The best type of patient is the patient that has already received great care from you practice before. They already know, like and trust you. Which means they are already sold on you, they just need to be offered something else that they want.

That's why you should spend just as much money marketing to get your past patients to come back to your practice as you do to people who've never shopped at your practice before. After all, your past patients are the ones who are the easiest to convince to come back to your practice and will be most willing to refer others to you.

So, you should also have specific marketing strategies that are designed to keep your past patients coming back to your practice in addition to getting new patients.

CHAPTER 5

New Patient Attraction Marketing Systems:
The Top Marketing Strategies That You Can Use To Consistently Fill Your Practice With More Patients

In this current economic environment, you have to do things strategically in order to have success in getting new patients. It's even more important now than ever before because things are not as easy as it used to be.

You must do things like offer more flexible financing and give substantial thought to how you are positioning your practice in your marketing and advertising.

More importantly, when you set out to implement anything in your practice, whether it is your collection system or the marketing system, you need to approach it as if you're setting up a system.

The Marketing Plan

At this point every doctor knows that having a marketing plan that you strategically implement is absolutely critical. However there's a common misconception that you can just grab a plug-n-play marketing plan and implement it into your practice. That's a huge mistake that many doctors make.

Don't Skip This Step

One of the important steps that will determine how successful your marketing plan will be is your ability to get your ideal target market to take action. The most effective way to do that is to target at least one specific type of patient for each marketing strategy you implement.

You may find this to be difficult because your first instinct will probably be to make each marketing strategy as broad as possible. However, your most effective marketing strategies will be the ones that speak to a specific target market.

Who Are You Marketing To?

There are five general groups of patients that come through the doors of your practice:

1. **Emergency/Event-Driven Type Patients** - Just want to be fixed.

2. **Reactive Patients Type Patients** - Know they should be getting treatment but have an excuse for not getting it.

3. **Proactive Type Patients** - Value a healthy lifestyle and participate in their preventative care.

4. **Discretionary/Optional Type Patients** - Just want to look or feel better, but no pressing issue.

5. **Regenerative Type Patients** - It's worth the investment to get a non-event driven outcome.

Emergency/Event Driven Patient

These are patients that primarily only visit when there is an event that forces them to get treatment at your practice. While all patients may require emergency treatment at some point, these types of patients are normally not active in your practice and only show up for emergency related services.

They don't call or come in until something significant happens. It might be that they're in pain, they have trauma, something broke or fell out.

Often, they have helped create the emergency through neglect. These patients tend to be very limited in their outlook and very resistant to hearing anything beyond their immediate perceived need.

The Event-Driven Patient Profile

There are several generalizations we know about this type of patient:

- May be overly fearful or phobic
- May be very limited financially
- May never have experienced regular care
- Not interested in a complete treatment plan
- No commitment to hygiene or periodic exams
- Accepts minimal care

To attract this type of patient with your marketing, you should focus on condition specific marketing strategies.

The Reactive Patient

These are patients who understand the need for regular follow-up and exams, but who for one reason or another only participate in a limited way.

They tend to float in and out of your practice from time to time whenever they have a small discomfort or concern that reminds them they haven't seen you in a while.

Then, after a couple of visits, they disappear again, until something prompts them to return. They go through these cycles because although they know what they should be doing, they haven't prioritized ongoing care enough so that it can compete with other demands and distractions life brings.

Reactive patients typically have a ton of excuses for not sticking to treatment plans, but these patients make up a significant "ground floor" of opportunity in the practice.

The Reactive Patient Profile

There are several generalizations we know about this type of patient:

- Understand the reason for ongoing care and periodic exams
- Participate in a limited way
- Sometimes return is prompted by concern or guilt
- Primarily accepts essential ongoing care
- Drops out of accepted treatment plan when fatigued

The Proactive Patient

These are patients who understand the value of a healthy lifestyle and participate in their preventative care. They are committed to regular preventative care and they regularly set appointments in advance and consistently follow-up.

However, a major concern for these patients is "cost." The economical impact of their ongoing care is a major factor and insurance is important to them.

These types of patients trust your diagnosis and they may be interested but they have to balance that against the age-old question: Is it worth it? This is the largest segment and essential "bread-and-butter" core of your patient base.

The Proactive Patient Profile

There are several generalizations we know about this type of patient:

- Understand the value of basic preventative care
- Participate regularly and follow-up consistently
- Insurance-driven in their decisions
- Typically complete treatment they accept
- Are often reluctant when it comes to more comprehensive care

The Discretionary Patient

This patient is the type of patient to look beyond essential and preventative care and make an investment in aesthetic treatment. It can be any number of perceived (or actual) defects that are bothering the patient but for whatever reason they've recently become larger than life in their minds.

While these patients often bring in the most revenue, they can also appear to be the most difficult to attract to your practice. Often these patients are proactive patients who have been influenced to take action by you or by an external motivator.

What Motivates These Patients?

The discretionary patient is usually a great patient to work with because they're so receptive. They are surprisingly open to everything that will help them reach their desired outcome. However, it's very difficult to consistently find this type of patient in your existing patient database because outside factors primarily influence them.

Things like a TV makeover show, a friend or coworker who is attractive, a new higher-profile job, an upcoming wedding etc. No matter how small or large the case, these patients now have a value mindset that is a breath of fresh air.

The Discretionary Patient Profile

There are several generalizations we know about this type of patient:

- Focused on appearance/correction of defects
- You often wait for them to self-identify
- Often influenced by outside sources (media, friends, new circumstances)
- It's not about insurance
- Interdependent care with specialists and lab
- Overall health may not be good

The Regenerative Patient

This type of patient is the best type of patient that you could hope to attract with your marketing. The regenerative patient is very aware of value beyond aesthetics and wants their outcome to be "as good as new" or even better.

They want the best that you have to offer: the highest contemporary standards using the best modern materials and techniques. In many ways they will challenge you because they often want you to push the envelope in an attempt to feel or look better than ever before.

That's an awesome goal but it's simply not always possible given the health and starting point of the patient. However they still have this desire.

The Regenerative Patient Profile

There are several generalizations we know about this type of patient:

- Highest level of care—as good, or better than nature
- Sometimes a "high discretionary" patient ("I want the best!")
- Sometimes a "high need" patient ("Is there any hope for me?")
- Usually doesn't matter where their health is now
- Interdependent care with specialists and lab

They All Need A Home

Now that we have a thorough understanding of these five types of patients and what drives them, you can strategically market to each. It should be crystal clear by now that each type of patient is driven and motivated by different factors. Those factors are what you are going to want to highlight in each of your advertising strategies.

On the other hand, if you've only focused on one type of patient in the past, then that explains why you might've gotten lackluster results. Going forward, you're going to have to speak to the goals and aspirations of each type of patient.

The Four Groups of Marketing Strategies

Once you have a good understanding of the types of patients you're going to be dealing with in your practice marketing, it's time to cover the four groups of marketing strategies.

Marketing Strategies #1: Internal Marketing Strategies

The first group of marketing strategies that you must implement in your practice is called internal marketing strategies. These are marketing strategies that get your existing patients to increase their average patient visit by either making new offers to them or encouraging them to complete their entire treatment plan.

Internal marketing strategies are so important because you need to know that you have systems in place to keep all of the new patients that you're attracting to your practice.

Marketing Strategies #2: External Marketing Strategies

The second group of marketing strategies is called external marketing strategies because they are all focused on strategies that attract new patients from outside your practice.

External marketing strategies are critical to your practice growth because without new patients, your practice will be limited in growth.

Marketing Strategies #3: Public Relation Marketing Strategies

The third group of marketing strategies is your public relations marketing strategies. These strategies are all about getting free publicity for your practice through several proven strategies to get local media to tout the best aspects of your practice.

Marketing Strategies #4: Online Marketing Strategies

The online marketing strategies probably hold the largest room for improvement so let's go in-depth.

The Great Leveler

A savvy doctor can dominate their target market with just a simple website, free Twitter account, free YouTube account and a free Facebook page. The Internet has leveled the playing field and opened up the door for the doctor with a small marketing budget to compete for a large market share.

Never in the history of the world has life-changing success for your practice be so easily accessible.

However, the true power isn't simply because a practice has a website or social media accounts on the Internet, it's about using your website, social media and the internet to get people to come into your practice.

Online Marketing Myths

Now although marketing online can dramatically change your practice, some doctors believe several myths about marketing online that are simply not true.

1. **Myth #1:** They believe that marketing online is too complicated and expensive for doctor's to do.

2. **Myth #2:** All you need is a website and you are guaranteed to instantly get tons of people to come to your practice. Nothing can be further from the truth.

3. **Myth #3:** They believe that you need to spend a fortune on a very expensive website to get people to visit their website and their practice. Fancy expensive websites that just look pretty will not help you.

4. **Myth #4:** If your website is on the first page of Google, then their practice will be flooded with patients. What matters more is how many people are going to your website and then taking action, like calling to schedule an appointment.

5. **Myth #5:** Marketing on the internet can solve all your advertising and marketing problems. Again, this is far from the truth.

6. **Myth #6:** All you need is a Facebook page and a twitter account and you'll automatically get more patients. That's another common misconception.

These myths are holding many doctors back from truly succeeding in their practices by using the power of the internet. However, even when doctors attempt to market their practice online, many still fail. Here are the major reasons why that happen.

Why 99% of Practice Owners Fail

1. They don't focus on the patients and prospects in their local market. Also known as local search – where people in your area are looking for solutions to their problem.

2. They don't have a major strategy to guide their actions. They just have a random set of marketing actions with no plan.

3. They don't understand how to create online marketing campaigns that drive people to their practice.

4. They don't tie their internet marketing actions and strategies with their traditional successful practice strategy systems.

5. They don't utilize marketing automation tools that make it easy to stay in front of past patients and get them back in the door.

6. They don't track results, so there's no way to know what is and isn't working.

Don't Ignore The Truth

In order to be successful with your online marketing efforts, you need to accept the truth about marketing your practice online. See, people love to talk online about their experience at your practice.

So, that means that people are now using social media sites like Facebook, Twitter and review sites like Google and Yelp to share their opinions of your practice online.

This means that your potential patients are also using these same places to see what other people are saying about you. You would have to be crazy to ignore these new trends.

Sit Up And Pay Attention

That's why it's important that you first setup, monitor and maintain your website, social media webpages and review websites. This is your basic online foundational footprint. The base components for how people find and get to know you.

At the end of the day, what others say about your practice, whether good or bad, has a big impact on whether potential patients will give your practice a shot.

However, if you don't update, monitor or maintain your online reputation and resources, you're going to lose out on hundreds and possibly thousands of potential patients.

Plus, it's also important for you to have a good grasp of online marketing so that you can track and monitor the results of your online marketing strategies. Let's talk about competition which is quite tough in this market.

Competition Is Fierce

As an independent practice owner, you are in a dogfight for patients when you market online because big conglomerates are many times more likely to provide all of the online things that your patients want.

Things like:

- More convenient hours and locations.
- Multi-discipline doctors in one central location.
- Attractive offer and prices.

To make matter worse, those behemoths are nearly ten times more likely to have a comprehensive online marketing plan than independent doctors.

That's why you have to have a game plan for turning tweets, posts and reviews into paying patients. You can't simply throw some stuff up and think it will work out okay.

Right In Your Backyard

See, most doctors want a website and a Facebook page so that they can become a big brand and be famous. But, it takes more than just a Facebook page and a few tweets here and there to get more patients your practice.

The fact of the matter is that there are more than enough patients within 5-10 miles of your practice to fuel a high six or seven figure practice for you. But that's only possible if you take the time to create a good plan to consistently market your practice online in your local area.

Just Another Tool

Many doctors get stressed out over how rapidly the internet changes and how they can best use it to promote their practice. The first thing you need to keep in mind about using the internet to grow your practice sales is that the internet is just a tool for you to use in your practice marketing toolbox.

Don't get overwhelmed by all of the options and new websites, software and programs that are coming out every day. You must have a simple plan that you create once, review each week and update about once per month and then stick to it. In other words, you need a plan that you consistently follow and implement.

Online Marketing Formula For Practices

The ideal plan for generating patients from the internet doesn't have to be complicated. However, you must follow a specific set of steps in order to do it successfully.

Here are the steps:

1. **You need to map out your process** – This includes mapping out your entire process for working with a prospect generated from any source on the internet.

2. **You need to identify your target prospect -** In order for any marketing or practice growth strategy to work, you have to first

know who you're trying to get or who you are trying to attract to your practice.

3. **You need to create your offer -** Once you attract prospects to your website or social media webpage, you need to have one or more compelling and persuasive offers to get them into your practice quickly.

4. **Attracting the prospects -** This is all about selecting online marketing strategies that gets your offer in front of your target prospects.

5. **Lead capture –** This is your method for getting prospects to give you their contact information in exchange of the offer or good that they are going to get.

6. **Cultivating your leads** – These are your tactics for building a relationship with your database of contacts over time in order to make your offer and then in order to get them into your practice quickly.

Follow The Plan

Following this proven blueprint eliminates the guesswork, confusion and dramatically eliminates the risk of major failure of your marketing efforts.

You will grow to love following up with the patients that are generated from your online marketing efforts because you have a proven blueprint to convert them into paying patients. More importantly, your patients will enjoy coming to your practice and will become raving fans.

And raving fans will be happy to tell others how wonderful you are.

CHAPTER 6

Telephone Call Mastery: The Proven System For Answering Your Phones That Quickly Turns Callers Into Paying Patients

In the large majority of practices, 95%-99% of the revenue is generated by a patient picking up a phone and calling the practice. That's why the fastest and most effective ways to increase the amount of new patients that flow into your practice involve your telephone.

Whether it be using different scripts or training and retraining your staff, the fact of the matter is that some of the biggest leaps in revenue will be a direct result of changing the way your staff handles incoming and outbound phone calls.

Are Your Phones Being Answered Correctly

Have you ever listened to how your front office people are answering your practice phone? Most doctors and practice owners haven't ever taken the time to record their phone calls so they have no idea what's happening in their front office.

Therefore it's never occurred to them that the person answering their phone might actually be STOPPING patients from setting appointments. It might not be intentional and they may not even realize their words on the phone are stopping callers from making or keeping their appointments. The worst part is that it can be totally preventable with just a few changes.

The Truth of The Matter

What your staff says to your callers on the phone plays a huge role in the caller making an appointment. That's why in order to have callers consistently booking appointments; incoming calls must be strategically answered to result in appointments.

Then, in the process, your staff finds out everything they can to help meet the needs of the person calling so that the person will keep that appointment.

This means that the person calling has not really been helped if they make no appointment and never actually gets to see you. The truth of the matter is when this happens the person answering the phone has actually stopped the caller from being helped in the best way possible.

Your Success Is In Their Hands

Before the patient sees you, they speak to the person you have entrusted to answer the phone, therefore you need to be able to answer the following questions about that person:

- Who is the person you have chosen to answer your phone?

- Do they know what to say and ask?

- Has anyone trained them to know what to say?

- Is anyone checking that they are saying the right things on the phone?

Sadly in most practices, the doctor doesn't have an answer to any of the questions I just asked. Even more surprising is the fact that even if they know the answers to the questions, they may still not know if what their staff are saying on the phone is the most effective.

Your Patients Are Valuable

In order to realize how important phone call mastery is, you and your staff must always be aware that every patient is worth over $2,000-$20,000+ to the practice. It's more than just the few hundred dollars you may get on their first visit.

Each patient is worth many multiples of that initial dollar amount. Especially when you factor in family, friends and other referrals they will generate.

So if your staff screws up the phone call, then you never get the chance to get their three or four family members and other valuable referrals. That's why you must focus on getting the patient into your practice. That's the only way you can generate revenue.

Shooting Yourself In The Foot?

When a patient calls in they are calling because they have a problem. One of the biggest mistake staff make is they try to screen out the patient over the phone.

Your staff shouldn't be asking or doing anything that discourages a person from setting an appointment and coming to your office. They shouldn't be asking them what kind of insurance they have or anything like that. Also, they shouldn't be asking questions about their age, gender, marital status or anything like that. You don't want there to be any hurdles in the way of new patients coming into your practice.

Telephone Call Master Basics

The Call Answering Basics

People don't call your practice at 9 pm at night expecting to talk to a live person. However, they do call during all times of day and early evening and expect a competent person to answer the phone, especially during the hours of 8:30 am - 6 pm.

However, most practices don't have someone to answer during lunch time and definitely don't have a live person until 6 pm in the evening.

So that means that for every hour that you don't have someone to answer the phone you are missing out on your chance to get new patients. This is a huge problem in the large majority of practices that must be addressed to increase the flow of new patients coming in.

There are even times when new patient inquiry calls are put on hold. New patients should never be put on hold except in extreme emergencies. Your staff shouldn't be trying to multi-task while on the phone with new patients.

There may even come a day where you need to hire a full-time person just to answer the phones for new patients. If you're currently at 50-60 new patients a month, then you should definitely have a dedicated phone team that is responsible for setting new patient appointments.

Keep in mind that your new patient phone call is your most important phone call in your office.

Do You Use Your USP On Phone Calls?

When new patients call your practice, does your staff say anything to them that sets you apart from the other offices they may have already called? If you're staff is saying the same old generic information that every other practice is saying, then something is wrong.

When the calls come in, your staff needs to ask or let the caller know something they did not know or thought about before. Your point of difference can be as simple as one or two questions to create curiosity and concern in the caller's mind.

- "How long have you had this discomfort?"

- "Have you had this before and then it went away?"

- "Does it wake you up at night?"

- "Is this something you have been wanting to get started with for a while?"

- "Is there anything else you are concerned about?"

- "Is there anything else you think I should know before we make your appointment?"

Be Brave And Standout

Most practices answer the phone in a pleasant and kind manner. You may think this is a point of difference but it really isn't. Most practices will talk to the caller with generic questions and answers that don't let the caller know that your practice is different.

Simply listening to the needs of the caller without trying to pre-qualify, disqualify or rush them off the phone can also be a big point of difference. Mostly because listening and finding out is really the only way to provide the best advice to then make the correct appointment for the caller.

If your staff can start the caller thinking differently about their issues by asking them better questions, then you will send the message to the caller that your practice has more expertise and you really know what you are doing.

What Does Your Staff Say?

Does your staff label callers and give them a name as to what type of patient they think they are before you really know them?

Most staff privately say things about your callers like:

- "That person was just a shopper"
- "They were not serious"
- "What a rude person"
- "They asked so many questions"
- "They sound like trouble"
- "They just won't listen to what is best"

Usually these comments are made after only a short time on the phone. Often the offending staff member doesn't even give the caller a chance. What do you think this does to the mindset and heart set of your staff if they are openly talking about your prospective new patients this way?

Get To The Heart of The Matter

You need to impress upon your staff that they are in the business of helping people and the only way to do that is to ask questions and listen with an open mind and heart. Once they actually listen, they may now start to understand why the patient has asked for the price or may have been a bit rude and abrupt.
Under no circumstances should your staff be quick to pre-judge your callers. That's why they need to take the time with each call to find out

about your caller. Instead of hanging up and calling them names, stay on the phone, find out what they need and make an appointment for them.

Patient Buying Signals

Most questions your staff will receive will be buying questions. Consequently, your staff must become fluent at understanding the difference between real objections and a buying signal.

Here are some examples of questions that patients ask right before they make a buying decision:

- How much does it cost?
- When are you open today?
- How do you handle this specific type of insurance?
- Are you taking new patients?
- Do you accept kids?
- What types of insurance do you accept?

8 Types of Calls

There are eight types of incoming calls into your practice and each call needs to have a process and system for being handled.

1. New Patients
2. Existing Patients
3. Vendors
4. Patients/People Trying To Pay You
5. Personal Calls
6. Other Doctors
7. Sales/Telemarketing Calls
8. Administrative

Call Prioritization

This step is to be mentally ready to answer every call and maximize that conversation. This starts by eliminating or dramatically minimizing personal phone calls. Your staff should never be afraid to put a non-wanted or pesky phone call on hold.

The top three important phone calls are: new patients, existing patients and people trying to make a payment. Your staff has to be able to get on and off the phone quickly and efficiently with everybody else.

You Don't Know What You Don't Know

Most doctors mistakenly believe that their front office team says the right things over the phone. Many even believe that they have a great team on the front desk because they've been at the practice for a long time.

The fact of the matter is that you can't possibly know what your staff is doing on the phones unless you record the calls and regularly listen to each recording.

You also need to know with precise accuracy the number of new patient enquiry calls and how many of those callers make appointments. Having these numbers is a measure of the success of the calls, lets you know how well the calls are going and enables you to decide if your front office really does need help.

You Have To Get To The "Why"

Many times when staff answers the phone, during the course of the conversation, they lose sight of the reason why the person calling has called in the first place.

In its most simplistic form, the new patient call comes down to these three things:

1. Listening carefully
2. Asking the right questions
3. Make the appointment

It's really that simple, but during the call several things derail that simple plan. First, when some staff members are asked one simple question, they may believe that gives them the green light to fire with tons of unasked for information.

Then because of the sheer volume of information, many callers are overwhelmed and go from wanting to be helped to just wanting to get off the phone as quickly as possible.

The way to avoid this is for the staff to answer the caller's very first question with a question of their own.

Don't Forget The Reason They're Calling!

The most effective calls are the ones where the staff is active listeners and the caller is doing most of the talking. The reason why this works best is because the person asking the questions and then listening is actually in control of the call and this is what you want.

After all, the first call as an opportunity to find out as much as you can about the caller; about their concerns as well as something personal about the caller themselves.

In order to do this, all your staff needs to do is ask another question appropriate to what you have now found out about the caller and then be an active listener again.

Then, they can just keep on doing this with questions leading them to the point where they feel you have listened and helped them and then set the appointment.

Getting New Patients To Show Up For Appointments

There is an art and science to getting patients to show up for their appointments. It basically boils down to this: You need to ALWAYS make sure the reason for that patient to keep their first appointment is greater after they finish the call than it was before they first called your office.

This means that your staff needs to become experts at increasing the level of concern that something bad, painful and possibly irreversible may happen if the new patient does not come in to see you as soon as possible.

While that may not be true in 100% of the cases for new patients, it's probably true in the large majority of cases.

Make Them Show Up For Appointments

In order to feel justified in encouraging callers to show up for appointments you have to acknowledge their reason for calling in the first place.

A potential new patient often calls for the following reasons:

- They have a medically related emergency.

- They are concerned about something with their health.

- They are not happy with something specific that's going on.

Ultimately, the reason for the call may be very urgent or it may not, but all callers have questions and your staff needs to be fluent in building causes for concern into their answers to those questions.

Don't Blow It

Many doctors cringe at the thought of increasing the level of concern for a caller, but if you want to help the most amount of people you must be able to get them to take action. Therefore without the building of concern and urgency, the caller will end the call and doubt their need to come in right away, if at all. This is when they often call back to cancel their appointment.

Answering their questions with other questions will create concern in their mind and will get the caller thinking. After all you really only have one opportunity to help them. It is your duty to make an appointment for them during this first call.

Can You Help Me?

In order to increase the caller's level of concern, you should have a list of great questions that will increase the caller's concern and urgency. You want to create doubt in the caller's mind so that they set and keep their appointment so they can get answers to their most pressing questions.

You want the caller to start to think about things they have not been thinking about. This will immediately create greater curiosity and concern in their mind.

As a result, the caller will have a greater desire to set and keep their appointment. They will have more questions they will want to ask which will make it much more likely that they'll keep their appointment.

Why Patients Cancel Appointments

There are four main reasons why a patient cancels their appointment or leave the practice without their next appointment.

1. Not enough urgency and concern was given to the patient before they left your office or over the phone.

2. You didn't find out if there was anything standing in the way of them getting started with their treatment. For example: fear, money, time, trust.

3. They didn't understand their treatment.

4. You did not build enough trust and belief in their treatment

Dealing With Last Minute Cancellations

One of the quickest ways to throw your day into upheaval is to have several last minute cancellations. That's why it's important to know how to handle this type of call but also important to stop it happening in the first place.

The fact of the matter is that there are really only TWO types of cancellations

1. The cancellation where the person just cannot come in for their appointment.

2. The cancellation where the person can change a few things to still keep their appointment.

Therefore the crux of the cancellation issue is can the staff member answering the cancellation phone call change the caller's mind?

Don't Encourage Cancellations

See if the person taking the last minute cancellation calls has the right strategies and skills, they can discourage the large majority of whim cancellations. However, most staff members simply say, "That's OK," when a patient calls at the last minute to cancel their appointment.

The worst part is that in most cases the staff reassures the person that it's okay to cancel before they even ask why there is a need to cancel that appointment.

Your perspective as the leader of your business is that it's not okay to cancel an appointment last minute for any reason under the sun. It needs to be a real emergency that can't be rescheduled.

Some practices go so far as to have a cancellation fee without a set amount of notice. This too can be an effective tool to put a stop to last minute cancellations.

Can I Change Your Mind?

You must communicate to your staff that it is NOT okay for scheduled patients to cancel for any reason they want.

Especially not when you have to meet your target for the day, other patients have missed out on this appointment time and the patient who has cancelled is not getting the treatment they really need today.

CHAPTER 7

New Patient Welcome System: How To Wow First-Time Patients And Make Them Fall In Love With Your Practice

In today's highly competitive business climate, the only practices that are thriving are the ones who realize they have to be very different from the other practices in their area. Your patients have hundreds of choices that are simply a click away, so if you're not doing something that's unique, you're essentially invisible.

Therefore if your patients can't easily distinguish the things that make you different, from the guy down the block, it's ONLY a matter of time before your entire practice begins sliding downhill.

By the way, "I liposuction better" or "I adjust backs better" or "I do something better" is NOT a difference ANY patient is ever going to realize.

The Big Lie

If you go to association meetings, or read the trade journals, they all tell you that the way to become more successful in your practice, is to upgrade or buy more expensive equipment or get more certifications, degrees or accreditations. However, that's not going to do one thing to make you more money or help you keep your existing patients or get them to spend more money with you, and refer more patients to you.

The reality is that being deeply committed, incredibly talented, and capable of caring for your patients is one thing. However creating a stable, predictable, and successful practice with abundant and consistent cash-flow coming in is completely different.

Obviously, I'm not suggesting you use old or inferior equipment or provide anything less than the best possible care. However, the truth is that patients don't care how much you "know," until they know how much you care.

The New Patient Experience Truth

Unless your patients are experiencing multiple unique caring "touch points" throughout their interaction with you and your team, then you're absolutely NO different from the practice down the street.

Contrary to popular belief, a unique new patient experience is a lot more than a few words on some brochures sitting in a rack in your waiting room. After all, the practice down the street also has those same brochures, plays soft music and bought new furniture and flooring to "jazz things up."

It's also more than putting your head down and working harder. After all, patients don't assume that working harder and caring are the same thing.

Besides if you only focus on working harder, then the amount of money you can earn will always be limited by the amount of time you're either willing, or are physically able to put in.

Let's Count The Ways...

There are a lot of missed opportunities in most practices when it comes to differentiating a practice based on how you handle those caring touch points:

- At the first scheduling call
- Call to confirm their appointment if it is scheduled more than 24 hours in advance
- At their actual first day visit

- On their call in the evening of their exam to confirm what you found

- On the confirmation call for their report of findings and spouse attendance

- At their actual report of findings

- On the call after their first treatment appointment to see how they feel

Those examples above are just for new patients with one visit under the belt! You have even more opportunities as they follow your treatment plan. By the way, the more "caring touches" you handle correctly with your patients, the better your patient retention will be.

Look At It This Way...

In order to improve your new patient experience, you need to look at your process from the patient's perspective from time they enter your door. The bad news is that 99% of practices in your field perform the same routine: Greet, meet and seat.

However, the good news is that 99% of all practices in your field perform the same routine! That's why the opportunity lies in your ability to script and design a "new" new patient experience that separates you from other practices.

The Big Picture

There are three specific goals that you need to build your improved new patient experience around:

1. Quickly and correctly determine what is causing the patient's problem.

2. Clearly explain what is causing their problems and the treatment recommended in a specific way that stimulates the patient not to just accept the recommended care but rather WANT the care.

3. Deliver the care so the patient's quality of life is improved.

Everything that you do should be designed to contribute towards those three goals. However, the problem is that most doctors are great at number one and three, but don't understand all the contributing factors that address number two.

When Your New Patient Experience Works

Creating a unique patient experience that stands out in our patients mind is a worthy goal that is deserving of time and planning. It can have a dramatic impact on the bottom line in your practice.

More importantly, patients often experience the following:

- They are happy and see you as helping them
- They have overcome their fears by embracing how healthcare in your specialty has evolved
- They want to have a healthy lifestyle
- They trust you and accept your recommendations
- They come back for follow up appointments
- They don't cancel, no-show, or arrive late
- They don't show up on your "high-maintenance" lists
- They value your services and pay promptly
- They respond promptly when contacted
- They want friends and family to experience your care

The New Patient Mindset That Makes The New Patient Experience So Important

The Harsh Reality

Most doctors are in denial about how their patients view them, their industry and their practice, however the patient's perspective is what matters most. Yes it's difficult to accept criticism about your life's work and crowning achievement, especially when it's given harshly.

However, in order to understand how to create an effective new patient experience system, you have to know how patients see your practice and what they do and do not want. That's your starting point and will give you proper perspective on many of the policies and processes in your practice.

What New Patients Hate!

There are many things that new patients hate when they are going for their appointment that you must be aware of.

- **Long wait to get an appointment.** There are legitimate reasons for longer wait times for many practices, but the large majority are a result of having untrained staff offering the wrong date options.

- **Long waits at the office.** Every patient hates long wait times in your office. That's why you have to address office efficiency and delegation in your practice.

- **Feeling rushed through their visit.** Patients can sense when you're in a hurry and are rushing them along. Therefore patients don't come back because they don't feel like you have time for them.

- **Having to repeat their story multiple times.** You should never make patients repeat or provide the same information over and over. You need to have a streamlined information sharing process that goes with the patient throughout your practice.

- **Lack of empathy.** You have to make sure that you authentically communicate that you care with your patients. This has been proven to make patients more willing to forgive other inconveniences.

- **Weak rapport.** Most patients feel that their relationship with their doctor can be better. However it requires you to take an honest look at how you build rapport with patients.

- **Unclear follow-up plans.** When a patient leaves your office, there can be no question about the next step for them. They should know exactly what the next step is.

- **Difficulty contacting their doctors between appointments.** There are a segment of your patients who desire to have a direct line to you to get their questions answered. Are you open to email access or direct call-in hours?

Here's What Patients Value

On the other hand, there are several things that patients value about the practice they choose:

- Prompt new patient exam
- Staff warm and helpful
- Highest standard of cleanliness
- Up to date facility and equipment
- Follow up phone calls
- Personal appearance and hygiene of staff and doctor
- Your staff doesn't look like late stage patients dealing with the same ailments you treat
- Practice hours
- Practice location
- Clearly explained treatment plans and financial options

Are You Easy To Work With?

Another contributing factor in a great patient experience is the ease in which patients feel when they go through your new patient process.

- Is your initial paperwork too long?
- Do you bring up the money and financing at the wrong time?
- Do you allow your patients to lose momentum by coming back the next day or two?
- Are you selling your treatment too aggressively?
- Are you over-educating your patients and taking way too long to do it?
- Are you regularly told that your first time visit is too high?

CHAPTER 8

Loyalty Marketing Systems:
How To Practically Guarantee That Your Patients Buy From You For Life!

The easiest patient to get into your practice is a past patient who already knows, likes and trusts you because they've received treatment from you before. Think about it: Who would you rather call or send a marketing message to? A past patient that has already purchased from you previously or someone you've never met, to whom you'll have to explain your product or service and convince them it's got value and that you are a trustworthy and reputable practice?

Satisfaction Is Nearly Worthless

In the good old days most doctors focused on satisfying their patients, but after hundreds of thousands of patients were surveyed, it was discovered that:

- Satisfied patients rarely refer anyone to a practice and often go to direct competitors of the practice they claim to be satisfied with.

- Loyal patients tell everyone about the practice without even being prompted AND stay with the practice they're loyal to.

- Loyal patients proactively look for other patients for you and encourage them to visit your practice.

So the moral of the story is that you want loyal patients who buy from you over and over. That's how you'll know they're satisfied.

That's why you should invest just as much money and resources in keeping your past patients as you do in getting new patients. In other words you should focus on creating patient loyalty in your practice.

The Patient Loyalty Advantage

A loyal patient is a patient that stays with your practice because they actually trust you and have a meaningful connection to your practice. They are loyal to your practice because your service is exceptional as the reality is there are likely dozens of practices where they can get treatment but they stay loyal because your service is exceptional.

They are loyal to you because they believe that they're receiving much more in value than the price they're paying. They are also loyal to you because they trust that when a problem comes up, you'll exceed their expectations in how you solve that problem. In short they trust you.

So, because they are loyal to you, they tell their friends, family members and even complete strangers about your practice because they want to introduce people to your great products and services.

Ultimately patient loyalty is the ultimate reward that you receive because you consistently provide above average service and you know how to resolve problems and issues at an exceptional level. However, never forget that patient loyalty is a behavior, activity or process. The patient must be consistently doing something (preferably buying something from you) to be considered loyal.

Loyalty Has Its Privileges

While the most obvious benefit to having fiercely loyal patients is the increase in sales and profits, there are dozens of other benefits like:

- They follow your treatment plans
- They give you valuable feedback in a non-threatening way to improve your practice
- They tend to interact in a more positive way with your staff, creating a better "vibe" in your practice

- They tend not to explode on you when simple little mistakes happen
- They're more responsive to your marketing efforts

The list goes on and on, but I'm going to share the top six benefits for you so that you know the immediate impact they'll have on your bottom line right away.

Loyal Patient Benefit #1:
You generate profit

Getting new patients is expensive. Most practices don't know their true patient acquisition costs because they have never added up all of the costs of getting new patients. Costs like paying staff, marketing agencies, advertising, website, marketing salaries, promotional items just to name a few.

See if you add up all of these expenses and divide the total by the number of new patients obtained during that period, you'll get the true cost of getting a new patient. If you were to do this exercise, what you'd likely find is that don't actually make a profit from a patient until they have been in to see you twice or perhaps even a third time. That's why loyalty generates most of the profits.

Loyal Patient Benefit #2:
They send you referrals

Patients who are delighted with your product or service can't wait to spread the word to colleagues or friends. That's why word of mouth is the least expensive and most cost-effective patient acquisition strategy. It can also be the most powerful because the relationships that the patient has with the people he refers foster an added level of trust for your practice.

This is especially true today. People share their best and worst experiences on Facebook, Twitter, Pinterest, Yelp, YouTube, and other social media networks or blogs—not just in writing, but also with photos and videos. This organic and unsolicited word-of-mouth referral from a loyal patient is worth its weight in gold.

Loyal Patient Benefit #3:
They're not as price sensitive.

Loyal patients are not only looking at the purchase price. They expect and want a great experience coupled with their service. Plus, it's been found that they are willing to pay a premium to get personal recognition and an individualized experience.

This allows you to charge a premium price for a premium experience, service and product. This also increases your profits exponentially because it allows you make more profit per patient visit with little to no increase in your costs.

It's also been proven that patients who pay a premium price often experience a higher level of satisfaction with their purchase purely based on the price they paid.

Loyal Patient Benefit #4:
They pay you on time

Loyal patients help your practice thrive by paying on time, which provides you with steady, stable and predictable cash flow. Your faithful patients love your practice, keep their appointments and pay when expected because they want to be in good standing. This allows you to count on a steady, predictable cash flow from which you can pay your expenses and subsequently reinvest in your practice.

There are many practices that have more money tied up in outstanding receivables than they have actually flowing into their coffers. If none of the other benefits of patient loyalty resonate with you, this should definitely be worth working towards build a loyalty-inducing practice.

Loyal Patient Benefit #5:
They become your competitive advantage

The increase in revenue that loyal patients bring to your practice allows you the cash flow to upgrade every area of your practice. Over time this advantage begins to compound and with the right amount of strategic planning and implementing you have happier employees, the best equipment and service offerings and better marketing. But it also means that you have the resources to enhance your product/service and patient experience even more.

Your goal is for you to ultimately reach a point where any potential or regular patient that comes in contact with your practice will notice the difference. This continuous improvement inevitably results in your practice taking market share away from your competitors.

Loyal Patient Benefit #6:
They are more forgiving of mistakes

Every doctor has been in a situation where any number of issues arose. Maybe it was the wait time, billing issues or treatment plan gone wrong. However, when you're dealing with a loyal patient they will be more likely to accept your apology and the "fix" and move on.

This usually happens because they look at your practice from the point of view of caring and trust, so as long as they're handled correctly, the mistakes have less significance.

In fact, it's these very mistakes and issues that give you a chance to demonstrate to your patients that you go above and beyond when issues come up. The speed and quality of your fix creates a "wow" factor and gives you a chance to turn a problem into a positive story for your testimonials and successes.

However, The Fact of The Matter Is…

Despite all the numerous benefits of creating loyal patients, most practices spend 100% of their marketing budget to only get new patients.

Then, once they get a new patient, they immediately divorce the patient and act as if they never existed. Instead practices should be working to develop a lasting and profitable relationship with the patient who has voted with the money.

Loyalty Doesn't Just Happen

Patient loyalty doesn't just happen by accident while you're going along the course of running your practice. In fact, it's been proven that a regular patient goes through several stages before they become loyal:

1. **Stage 1: Suspect** - A suspect is anyone who might possibly become a patient at your practice. We call them suspects because we believe, or "suspect," they might be future patient, but we don't know enough yet to be sure.

2. **Stage 2: Prospect** - A prospect is someone who has a need for a procedure or treatment that your practice offers and is able to buy. Although a prospect has not yet purchased from you, he may have heard about you, read about you or had someone recommend you to him. Prospects may know who you are, where you are and what you sell, but they still haven't bought from you.

3. **Stage 3: Disqualified Prospects -** Disqualified prospects are those prospects that do not need, or do not have the ability to pay for treatment or procedures at your practice.

4. **Stage 4: First-Time Patient -** A first-time patient is someone who's been treated at your practice at least one time.

5. **Stage 5: Repeat Patient -** Repeat patients are people who have been treated at your practice multiple times.

6. **Stage 6: Advocate -** An advocate is a patient who is constantly being treated at your practice because they either have an ongoing condition, long-term treatment plan or they are seeking help in reaching a desired outcome. In addition an advocate encourages others to come to your practice. They talk about you, do your marketing for you and bring other patients to you.

Laws Of Building Patient Loyalty

There are several important practice principles that you need to be aware of that will determine how successful you can become at building patient loyalty in your practice:

1. **Focus on building staff loyalty** - Loyal patients want relationships and familiarity. They want to buy from people who know them and their preferences. It's virtually impossible to build strong patient loyalty with a high rate of staff turnover.

2. **Know where the money comes from** - All patients are not created equal. Roughly speaking, 80% of your revenue is being generated by 20% of your patients. Some patients spend more and thus they represent more long-term value to your practice than other patients. That's why you need to pay super close attention to the high-value patients.

3. **Know the loyalty stages** - Patients become loyal to a practice and its products and service one step at a time. By understanding the patient's current loyalty stage, you can better determine what's necessary to move that patient to the next level.

4. **You must present options to them** - Today's patients are smarter, better informed and more intolerant of "being sold and/or told" than ever before. They expect to be presented with options that are clearly explained in terms of procedure, cost and time.

5. **Look for patient** complaints - In most practice's 90% of patient complaints are unarticulated and manifest themselves in many negative ways like: unpaid invoices, lack of courtesy to staff, etc. You need to make it easy for patients to complain, and then take those complaints seriously by addressing them and fixing them.

6. **Be available for your patients** - Patients associate your responsiveness and availability to their perception of good service. Technology tools such as patient self-service, email management and live chat/Web callback are becoming mandatory.

7. **See your value from patients'** perspective - Knowing how your patients experience value and then delivering on those terms is critical to building strong patient loyalty. Keep in mind that patients' value definitions are constantly changing. That's why you must stay tuned in to your patients.

8. **Win back lost patients** - The average practice loses 20-40% of its
    patients every year, which is why it's important that you have a
    strategy for getting your past loyal patients to come back to you.
    After all, research shows that a practice is twice as likely to
    successfully sell to a lost patient as to a new prospect.

Having loyal patients has numerous benefits, however the sad reality is
that not every practice doesn't deserve loyal patients. See your
worthiness to expect loyalty depends on your ability to consistently
meet and exceed your patients' expectations.

Most practices have no problem meeting the bare minimum standard
that patients use to make a purchase decision. However, very few
practices exceed those minimum standards. That's why you need to
honestly evaluate how your practice is interacting and engaging with
your patients. You can get the best information by either secretly
shopping your own practice or hire a mystery shopper to get an honest
perspective from your patients view point.

Standout Or Sit Down

Standout patient service is the foundation upon which you build
your patient loyalty. No standout patient service = no widespread
patient loyalty. When you view every patient interaction as critical to
building patient loyalty, it instantly makes clear what the correct solution
to the situation should be. But at the end of the day, it is your level of
patient service—the way your practice treats and values patients.

Also, it's nearly impossible to talk about patient loyalty without talking
about patient service. All doctors know that without patients they don't
have a practice which is why they spend so much money to get patients.

However, their practice systems and processes don't always reflect a
"patient first" mentality. That doesn't mean the patient is always right,
but it means that you'll always do right by your patients because they
ultimately determine your success.

CHAPTER 9

Patient Referral Systems: How To Easily Get Local Businesses, Practices And Patients To Refer Their Family, Friends And Co-Workers To Your Practice

Patients who come to your practice as referrals from existing patients are more loyal, better prepared, and longer-term patients than those who become patients through coupons or loss-leader efforts.

Referrals are the best way to build a thriving practice and you should do everything in your power to consistently get them. However, like most successful practice building strategies, it takes real work and real changes, so many practice owners put it off.

In fact, 99.9% of doctors don't have a single system in place to generate referrals to their practice. You should have systems in place to get referrals from other practices, past patients and other local businesses or organizations.

Missing The Boat

Getting referrals is great because you can get hundreds of people to visit your practice at little to no additional cost. Plus, it's less expensive to generate referrals from existing patients than trying to get new patients. Referrals don't have to be convinced to come to your practice because they've already been pre-sold on coming, by other patients. When you create a referral marketing system, you partner with your past patients, other practices and local businesses, but you also create an awesome patient environment that builds patient royalty.

Beautiful Patient Referral Systems

There are many reasons why you need patient referral systems in your practice, but let's just look at a few:

- **They are systematic:** This means that the referral program can be replicated over and over again with the same or better results. The best referral systems keep on generating referrals month after month!

- **They work on a one-to-many basis:** High performance referral systems get multiple patients to refer your office simultaneously through the many referral campaigns that are generated from it!

- **They have the ability to tap into people's networks:** Transformational referral systems tap deep into the network of friends, family, and co-workers that your patients know!

- **They use incentives to motivate people to refer:** Let's face it, most people are either lazy or too busy to care about your office so the best referral systems use an incentive system to keep the referrals flowing.

Why Most Practices Are Not Worthy Of Receiving Referrals

While there are many benefits to developing systems to generate referrals, you must first make sure your practice is poised for success. Here are some of the reasons why many practices are not positioned for success when it comes to generating referrals:

- They have no real commitment to getting referrals

- There's too much focus on selfish reasons

- They don't even remember to ask for referrals

- They are really not doing something unique or different that patients can recommend to other people

- Assuming that a great service alone is enough

- Being afraid of asking for referrals

Three Types of Referrals Systems

There are three types of referral systems that you will need to have in place in your practice in order to systematically and consistently generate referrals:

1. **Current Patients:** Your existing active patients.

2. **Medical Practices:** Practices that have sent referrals to you before or that you want to send referrals to your practice.

3. **Local Businesses:** Businesses and organizations that you form strategic marketing alliances with. ie. Chamber of commerce, YMCA etc.

Referral System #1:
Patient Referral Generating System That Generates
Referrals From Your Current Active Patients

Patient Referral System

The first source of referrals you should focus on generating is from your past patients. If you're running a good practice, then this can be a goldmine. You always want your patient referral program to be a win-win. This means that you recognize and thank the patient who's referring and reward the referral for coming in to your practice.

The first step is that your current patient who's doing the referring can receive a personal handwritten thank you note or a personal phone call from your office. Meanwhile the patient that they referred can also receive a reward when they take you up on the irresistible offer that you put together for referred patients.

Patient Referral Basics

The first step in generating referrals is to start by letting your current patients know that you have openings for new patients. If you always look super busy to the patient they don't think to refer. Brochures or signs are helpful as reinforcement tools, but they are passive reminders and don't engage or inspire the patient directly.

Most doctors are too uncomfortable asking for referrals so simply letting the patient know that you are accepting new patients is a non-threatening way to plant the referral seed.

So start with something simple and easy to do like letting all of their current patients know that they're "now accepting new patients."

The good thing about using that simple statement is that it doesn't sound cheesy or contrived. It's just an honest little statement that rings true to both you and the patient. Also if you couple that with two or three referral cards, you have just created a simple little system that can generate five to ten new patients a month.

Referral System #2:
How To Consistently Generate
Referrals From Other Practices

When it comes to generating referrals from other practices, doctors need to like, trust, feel that you are competent and believe you are successful. In other words, you need to have a real relationship which requires time and attention to maintain and grow.

They want to be confident that the referral they make will be beneficial to their patients care, and reflect well on themselves. Professionals will refer with confidence when there is a strong and reliable relationship in place.

Relationship building begins by reaching out to your potential referral sources to learn how and if you can serve their needs. After you've listened, you can begin to educate them about your practice and how you can deliver the kind of patient care they value most.

Regardless of the type of referral providers you're targeting, there are some common threads that dictate their expectations for their referral partners.

- **High quality care:** You must have a well-established reputation for treating your patients with respect, taking time to answer their questions, and checking up on them after treatment. This shows that you truly care.

- **Timely appointments:** Make a special effort to accommodate the referred patient as soon as possible (and see them quickly once they arrive at your office).

- **Prompt understandable reports:** Let the referring practice know when the patient has been scheduled, that you appreciate the referral and that you will continue to communicate about what follows.

Referral System #3:
How To Build Your Practice Referral Generating System
That Gets Referrals From Local Businesses
(aka. Strategic Marketing Alliances)

When two practices work together to create a joint marketing campaign that benefits or drives patient growth to both practices, it's called a strategic marketing alliance. This can be done by mailing out letters of recommendations or endorsements to each other's patients and prospects.

But, it can also be something as simple as handing out coupons or vouchers to their own patients which will then encourage the patient to visit the practice of their strategic marketing partner. Regardless of the specific strategy used, the principle is that two different practices are helping each other to become more successful.

The Bigfoot of Practices

Strategic alliances are very effective ways of getting patients on a consistent basis, but this strategy does require you to step outside of your comfort zone in order to pull it off. That's why 99.9% of doctors don't even try to use this powerful practice building strategy.

However, don't dismiss it as being too hard, because it's so powerful that it can single-handedly transform your struggling practice into a success. That's why it's one of the best ways for you to drive tons of your ideal patients to your practice every day of the week.

Why Are Strategic Marketing Alliances So Powerful?

Strategic marketing alliances are one of the most powerful strategies you can get involved in because of seven reasons:

1. You will build a list of targeted patients and prospects that are most likely to visit your practice.

2. If done right, you will profit every time you form a strategic alliance while also building your list.

3. Your partnerships are a good way to build great relationships with other doctors in your community that will pay off for years to come.

4. There's little to no advertising or additional marketing expense to get these patients to come into your practice.

5. You can get access to a list of paying patients where someone else has already done the hard work.

6. It's easier to please these patients because you come highly recommended from a trusted source of theirs.

7. Using strategic alliances allows you to instantly position yourself as the best practice because you're coming recommended from a trusted practice.

The Strategic Alliance Mindset

When it comes to setting up strategic marketing alliances, you need to make sure that your motives are pure. You need to approach this from a win-win perspective and not come across desperate or sleazy. You need to authentically come across as someone who is genuinely adding value to your strategic marketing partner.

If you are blowing smoke, people can tell. However, if you're thrilled and enthusiastic, it will show and can have a positive impact on your potential partnership. That's why you need to come up with at least three to five things that partnering with you will help accomplish for your strategic marketing alliance partner in their practice.

Imagine

Imagine you find five strategic marketing partners that each have a list of 1,000 people. By partnering with them, you've now just become the practice of choice for 5,000 quality referrals from other practices... with NO extra advertising cost!

Word Of Caution...

On the other hand, the wrong strategic marketing alliance can do massive damage to your practice's reputation. That's why you must have systems in place to consistently deliver good food and a good experience.

So, if you're not ready to handle the influx of patients, then don't do it. Also, you need to be prepared to give more than you're getting to make the strategic alliance attractive. And you need to have several ideas to make a success for your alliance partner and your referrals.

All The Way To The Finish Line...

Even after you've set up a strategic marketing alliance, you need to stay on top of things to make sure your partner doesn't drop the ball. You should find a reason to stop by, email or call them to update them and let them know you're available if they have any questions.

You need to stay positive even if you're not seeing any results at first. Sometimes it takes a few weeks or even a few months for things to come together just right. Just be sure to get your partner to agree to a specific timeline for things to be completed to avoid any potential issues. If they start to lag, jump in and ask if there's anything you can do to help.

CHAPTER 10

Patient Marketing Systems:
How To Consistently Generate More Patient Visits From Your In-House Database

By now you already know that building your own in-house database of patients, prospects and past patients is critical. Now I want to teach you the most effective and profitable ways to follow up with your database of prospects and patients and get them to back into your practice time and time again.

Following up with your database or nurturing your patients consistently is your new philosophy that you must whole-heartedly adopt in your practice to be successful. However, it's more than just sending sales messages. Your goal is to own the space in your patients mind for the procedures, treatment plans and services that you offer.

See the truth is prospects and patients always forget about your practice over time. No matter how great the connection at the time a patient contacts or visits your practice, the longer you wait to follow up with them, the more they forget you.

That's why your mission is to build relationships with qualified prospects regardless of their timing to buy, with the goal of earning their business when they are ready to buy.

You accomplish this by consistently presenting the prospect with a persuasive sales message or educational message that compels them to visit your practice and buy. You want them to feel as if they MUST come to ONLY your practice when they're ready to buy AND when they're looking for information prior to buying.

Profitable Relationships

Follow-up marketing (also known as patient nurturing) is all about building a consensual relationship with a prospect—you can't force someone to commit (to a purchase, in this case)—but you also cannot afford to lose individuals because they're not ready to move forward today.

Most patients will eventually be ready, but it is up to you to both provide them with relevant information and to be there when they are ready to make a final decision.

Missing The Point

It's been tested and proven that it takes anywhere from seven to ten follow-up contacts or messages for most people before they will even consider doing business with you. However, most doctors don't do any follow up and if they do, it is usually one, or if they are really good, two. Do you see the problem?

Most doctors don't understand that if you do a presentation and the person does not elect to start treatment right away, it is not the end of your relationship—it is the beginning of your relationship.

Think about this. You test drive a new car or take a tour of a new home if you are in the market. When are you most likely to actually buy the car or buy the new home? Chances are that you are most likely a buyer within the first 30 days. That is the reason the salesperson or the real estate agent starts to follow-up with you right away. You need to do the same thing in your practice.

Tying Your Own Hands

The lack of follow-up literally throws away future cases that would have eventually gone forward. Those people that you're not following up with are still spending thousands of dollars with practices in your local area every single day. It's just not at your practice. The only real question is will they invest those dollars with your practice or the practice down the street.

If the average lifetime value of a patient in your practice is $1,500, do you think that it is a very good idea to keep in touch with EVERYONE that responds to your marketing message, knowing that once they are ready to buy they will very likely buy from you because you kept in contact with them? Hopefully your answer is yes!

Where Did All The Patients Go?

There are basically seven reasons that patients disappear and never show up to your practice again:

- **Reason #1 -** You got them better. A positive patient outcome.

- **Reason #2** - They chose pain relief and you delivered the goods. A positive patient outcome.

- **Reason #3** - You educated them or maybe you didn't and they are not sure they need to be there.

- **Reason #4** - Time became an issue for the patient.

- **Reason #5** - You dismissed them. Maybe they ran out of insurance, or they were a personal Injury or Workmen Compensation case. Whatever the reason you decided to dismiss them.

- **Reason #6** - They owe you money. This patient is not coming back. They are going to find another doctor they can owe money to.

- **Reason #7** - You didn't deliver the goods. Although it is rare, let's face it not every patient gets better and a few may even get worse. They are not coming back.

In the cases where patients experience positive outcomes, if they are not coming back to you it's because you are not keeping your name in front of your patients.

Just remember that if your name is always in front of your patients you won't have to figure out how to reactivate them, they will reactivate themselves.

Poised For Long Term Success

Building a list of past patients and prospects that you can market your practice to "on-demand" is your insurance policy against the revenue roller coaster most doctors have to endure.

Your database should be filled with thousands of patients, prospects and past patients who you can email, call or mail an offer to any time that you choose. Imagine the power of sending out an email, text, postcard or letter on Tuesday and being booked solid or flooded with patients for the next two weeks from that one marketing effort. That's powerful!

However, the reality is that most doctors do the opposite. They spend thousands of dollars each month trying to get the attention of a small percentage of people who may possibly be ready to buy today, but do little to keep in contact with people who have already purchased from them and/or raised their hand in some way to say they're interested in what they're selling.

The Big Mistake

While the most successful doctors that run thriving practices know that they must consistently follow up with their patients and prospects, struggling practices do the following:

- Look at ongoing marketing to their past patients and patients as an expense instead of an investment.

- They are not willing to take the time away from their practice to create a multi-step campaign that runs consistently.

- Are so busy working in their practice that they don't have time to work on their practice and create systems that will generate a huge increase in profits.

- Don't know and refuse to learn how to write educational, entertaining and persuasive marketing sales messages.

- Get overwhelmed by the technology required to setup automated follow-up marketing systems.

Most Common Excuses

Unfortunately many doctors know the benefits of follow up marketing, but they allow themselves to buy into excuses that hold them back from getting the most lucrative type of patient back into their practice.

The most common excuses are:

- Can't afford to pay for marketing to their database
- Don't have their patients or prospect's information
- Even if they had their contact details, don't know what to say
- Don't know how to contact the patients or patients
- Already have one million things going on right now
- Don't have someone to do this for them
- It seems too complicated
- Don't want to learn to use any more technology

Secrets To Follow-Up Marketing Success

In this section, I want to share with you the most powerful secrets that will allow you to experience massive success when you setup and implement your follow up marketing strategies.

Follow Up Marketing Success Secret #1:

The first follow up marketing success secret is to completely understand the buyers in your target market. You need to interview and survey your patients, as well as talk to those that didn't choose your practice, in order to define your ideal patient profile and develop buyer personas. You should ask questions like:

- What are their pains? What are their desires?
- What is their purchase process?
- Why were they interested in your service in the first place?
- What were the major factors in their purchasing decision?
- What else do you they want from your practice?

Follow Up Marketing Success Secret #2:

The second follow up marketing success secret is pinpointing and knowing the buying stage cycles for each of your procedures, treatment plans or services. This is so important because in order to create a follow-up marketing and nurture campaign that works you must consistently deliver timely and relevant information to your prospects. If the information is too late, too soon or not relevant, it won't work.

You need to know and fully understand those stages and what works best with each. All buyers go through these three stages:

The Buying Stage Cycles

1. **Stage #1: Just Started Looking:** To get these prospects to come and buy from you need to have things like: Free whitepapers, free books, free guides & tip sheets, free eBooks, free checklists, free videos, free kits and any combination of the above.

2. **Stage #2: Already Looking, But Need More Information:** You need to offer things like free webinars & teleseminars, case studies, free product or service sample, frequently asked questions sheet requests, product spec sheets, catalogs etc.

3. **Stage #3: Ready To Buy Now:** You want things like free trials, demos, free consultations, estimates or quotes, coupons etc.

Follow Up Marketing Success Secret #3

This success secret is all about analyzing your past marketing campaigns in order to determine how they contributed to revenue. You'll look at the percentage of responses to campaigns and determine how many patients moved through all stages, and the messages and content offered at each stage.

You should have a folder and binder (physical or on a computer) with every ad, promotion and sale you've ever run and the results of each. Otherwise how will you know what worked and how you can improve upon it? Reviewing the success (or failure) of your past marketing efforts is the foundation upon which you build your follow-up campaigns.

Follow Up Marketing Success Secret #4

This success secret is about visually mapping out the ideal new patient path for each of your core procedures, treatment plans and services. You should have a piece of paper(s) where you've mapped out your follow up marketing campaigns that essentially mirrors your actual in-practice process.

The key to mapping this out is to start out with the end goal in mind and create a roadmap that is specifically designed to get a prospect to that end goal.

Be sure to develop a roadmap that makes the most sense for your practice and try to anticipate any roadblocks to implementing it and address them early. If the objective is to send six emails and make three phone calls over eight weeks, what happens if you don't get the intended response after you do that? You need to have a plan for that too.

Follow Up Marketing Success Secret #5

This follow up success secret is all about automating your entire follow-up campaigns as much as possible. You already have enough on your plate to worry about. You don't want to have to manually send every email, lick every envelope, print every postcard etc.

Your follow-up campaigns must be able to be 99% automated with little human interaction needed to deploy or maintain the campaigns. An automated "welcome campaign" is a great place to get started. Set up automated communications to greet those who enter your database and start delivering educational information right away.

There are over ten follow-up marketing campaigns you can and should implement in your practice right away. Yes, setting up these campaigns sounds like a lot of work, although it really isn't, but the trade-off is HUGE for your profits bottom line. Do the work once and profit from it for years to come.

Is Your Practice Being Left Behind?

Now, if you fall into the category of practices that are not proactively working with these technology changes and marketing systems, **you are only going to see things get worse over time**.

These changes, though recent, are now a permanent part of the competitive landscape.

The gap between the practices that "get it" and those that don't is widening at an accelerating pace.

You can look at any industry and see examples of the handful of businesses that are really pulling away from the pack, and those that are falling behind.

It's Time to Go All-In

Do you have someone that is helping your practice in these areas?

Or are you kidding yourself into thinking that you are going to try to do this by yourself or with the very part-time effort of one of your employees that has no marketing background?

That's not going to cut it!

If you're struggling to fit everything into your calendar already (most practice owners I talk to are), you're probably not going to have the bandwidth to optimize all 8 of these profit boosting systems.

Either something else has to give, or you need to enlist a friendly expert to help you!

If You Are Ready to Make a Shift …

You may realize that you need to make a change, that you aren't growing like you should, that your current approach to marketing is not working, and that you are committed to getting past your current income limits.

If so, I would be interested in talking with you to see if there is potentially a good fit to work together.

However, I must say upfront that I only work with one client in your industry per city so I can give them all of my knowledge and experience without having to worry about conflict with another client.

And we are particular about who we work with. We only work with practices that are already successful and are looking for strategic ways to get FAR MORE successful.

We work with clients that have the mindset and resources to handle the level of growth that is possible to achieve.

What to Do Next

If you've seen the benefit of what you've read in these pages and you decide you'd like some assistance so you can focus on running your practice instead of all the tasks involved in marketing it, let me know.

We can take a close look at how your practice is doing now, what's needed to improve your systems, and how we can reach your goals together. No sales pitch… just solid information you can use to reach the next level.

Reach Out to Me Today

Jon Nare
Founder, True Inspired Solutions
Email: Jon@TrueInspiredSolutions.com
Phone: 480-331-8783

About the Author

Jon Nare is a founding partner in True Inspired Solutions where he helps cosmetic surgeons identify the biggest problems facing their practice in the areas of getting new patients, getting referrals, and getting repeat patients.

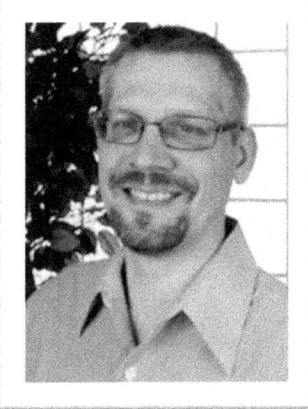

He then helps implement an action plan that automates getting more new patients, more referrals, and more repeat patients.

The result is explosive revenue and profits, in some cases double or even triple in as little as 90 days.

When not helping cosmetic practices, he can be found spending quality time with his loving wife, four children, and two grandchildren.

More details about Jon Nare can be found by going to his LinkedIn profile at:
>> TrueInspiredSolutions.com/linkedin/

www.ingramcontent.com/pod-product-compliance
Lightning Source LLC
Chambersburg PA
CBHW070809180526
45168CB00002B/542